I Was Healthy Until the Day I Wasn't

The Faces of Cancer

Jim Parise

outskirts
press

DEDICATION

This book is dedicated to all those whose lives became accidentally entwined with mine, whose faces have been indelibly etched in my mind's eye and whose courage and strength have become part of my every day life.

…to those who are still struggling with this disease and whose determination to survive has never flagged. Meryl, your strength inspires me. Jim M., you got this. Jason, you are a fighter. Lee, my fellow warrior. Sue D., for your survival. Ray, enough is enough. Darren, no three putts.

…to those who have lost the battle, you are with me, and you are in part, the motivation for writing this book. Sue, Matt, Truman, Des, Lew, my cousin Barbara A. and Terry forever in my heart.

…to the doctors, nurses and hospital staffs who work tirelessly in the face of adversity, putting aside personal issues to minister to our needs, I am indebted.

…And lastly to the caretakers. You are the unsung heroes of this disease. Often overlooked and eclipsed by the patient's illness, you exhibit heroism in times when there was nothing you could do to ease the suffering. You stood strong and carried us through when we were too weak to carry ourselves.

ACKNOWLEDGEMENTS

The following people need to be recognized and thanked for helping me through the healing process:

…to all those who drove me to appointments, sat with me through infusions and would not let me fall through the cracks, who took me to dinner or brought me meals: Ray and Sue L, Bob and Lenore D., Tom and Barbara S, Marilyn J., Brian and Lou J., Charlie and Sue D.

…to Dr. Christopher Pennell whose knowledge, experience and guidance contributed to my understanding of this disease and who metaphorically held my hand in the initial stages of questioning and decision-making

…to those who came to visit me in Hope Lodge, kept me company and had a meal with me so I would not have to eat alone: George and Kathy L, John H, Jen G, Joe R, (who dazzled Hope Lodge residents with his piano playing in the lounge), and Flo and Joe L.

…to all those who sent cards and notes to cheer me. Ginny M. you are the best.

… to Dr. Ken Fishberger and his office staff, in particular, Anna, who saw my helplessness and immobility and steered the direction my life was to take in the foreseeable future. You thought for me when I could not think for myself. Your kindness will never be forgotten.

… to Dr. Miguel Perales and the whole bone marrow transplant team for enabling me to walk my daughter down the aisle and witness the birth of my third grandchild. These gifts are the true blessings of my life.

…to Dr. Charles Davenport who guided and coaxed me to this point without judgment and always with kindness and understanding. You helped me process all of this, something I was unable to do on my own. Your encouragement brought me back to this project after a long absence.

FOREWORD

There have been many books written about cancer by patients or their caregivers. I have never read any of them. I knew what they said by reading about them or listening to interviews with the authors.

I did not know how to approach this. I wanted to find a new take on writing about cancer and not fall into a mundane treatment of the subject. I wanted to write a book about my journey (an already overused word in the life of a cancer patient and one I tend to use more than I should) and not have it fall into the realm of "been there, read that".

I kept thinking about it and nothing came to me. Being in isolation for nearly 70 days in a 20x20 room, with a miniature TV and not much else to distract me or help me pass the time, I resorted to setting up a blog, not only to chronicle my "adventures" and keep a time line for future reference, but also to field questions that were becoming overwhelming for my family and somewhat lighten the burden of their having to answer the same questions multiple times. I hoped that in doing this I could be honest and faithful to my experiences, throw in a little humor (ok, sarcasm too) and introduce the reader to the people I have met along the way.

Are my experiences any different or more valid than anyone else who has been stricken with this insidious disease? Maybe different but certainly not more valid. In your hands you are holding the story of those people and places and circumstances that have changed my life and now you are reading this. I hope that its straightforwardness might bring some understanding to those of you who have mercifully never been touched by cancer; a different insight to those who have a loved one who has; a commonality and a little humor to those of you who have faced this monster and have beaten it down for three months or three years or forever… is there such a word as "forever" in the world of cancer treatment? Do I dare use it? I do.

For Nancy, my fiancée at the time, who endured so much of this with me, but who took the time to nurture herself so she could be there for me, I am eternally grateful.

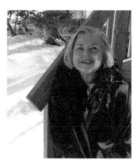

Nancy

For my sisters Susan and Laurie and their husbands, Don and Arthur, who stepped up to the plate and relieved Nancy of so much of her burden; who comforted me with laughter and homemade meals and crossword puzzles, and smuggled contraband wine into my room; and who facilitated the business and mechanics of my care, thank you all.

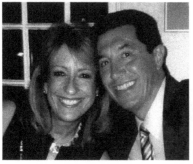 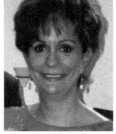 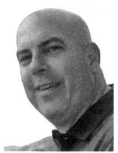

Susan and Don   **Laurie and Arthur**

For my children, Kristen and Jamie, who remained on the periphery for so long (I suppose out of fear) but who were always there with good intentions and private prayers. Good news, girls, you can take down the post-a-notes you put on my possessions to "mark your territory" — Daddy ain't gone quite yet.

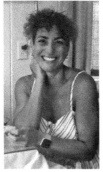

Kristen

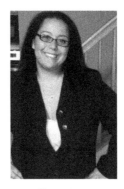

Jamie

And lastly for my grandchildren, Sophia and Mykayla. My thoughts of you, your youth and optimism, carried me through many of my darkest moments and strengthened my resolve to live long enough to see both of you into adulthood. And my newest granddaughter, Stella, who was not yet born, today you make Poppa laugh and keep his mind from wandering into dangerous places.

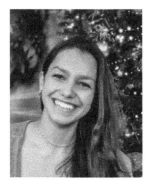

Sophia

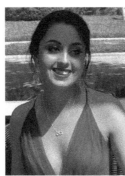

Mykayla

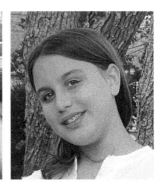

Stella

PART I

Chapter 1

Let's start at the very beginning —
December 6, 2006

The dull, muted sounds of the intercom paging Dr. So-and-So made it near-on impossible to get any sleep, even with the morphine trying its damnedest to offset the pain. Shadows moved about quickly, in stealth, past the emergency room bay, creating a strobe-like effect as they passed by the door, blocking the light from the hallway momentarily. And then gone, only to be followed in rapid succession by yet another silhouetted figure and another. The room went black again but stayed darkened this time as this large frame blocked nearly the entire doorway creating a halo-like effect around it. A nurse's gentle hand jostled my shoulder to wake me and as the figure from the doorway moved toward me, the light from behind it stabbed my eyes. "Mr. Parise, our preliminary tests show that you either have an infection, leukemia or cancer."

"What?" I replied groggily trying to come out of the stupor and adjust to the now bright fluorescents. The repeated diagnosis did little to clarify the onrush of thoughts and images that now crashed their way into my still fogged brain. "Herbie casts one vote for infection," I said, struggling to sit up. "Give me an antibiotic and get me out of here."

"It's not as simple as that. We have to run more tests. I've scheduled an oncological consult with a surgeon in the morning and he'll do a biopsy after he speaks with you," the ER physician said.

At 4 A. M., dulled by multiple morphine injections, even I knew that the words oncology, surgeon, biopsy used in the same sentence boded more than an infection. I closed my eyes and drifted into a fitful sleep. Alone, afraid and still trying to deny the pain in my gut was anything more than overeating and drinking during the holidays, I wept. I don't know what the young man who shared my ER bay thought of this old man convulsed by muffled sobs in the next bed was told but he averted my eyes when I looked at him as if to say, "What are you staring at? I've just been diagnosed with cancer, leukemia or an infection. What's your problem?" But he didn't look back at me. And then I slept.

When morning broke the nurse who had tried to comfort me, both physically and emotionally, awakened me. Her gentle manner strongly contrasted how rude and abrupt the doctor who followed her was. Two more faces. I began to realize there would be more like these opposites to follow. The oncological surgeon arrived for the "consult". Not sure why it's called a consult. No one had consulted me. I was just told what was going to happen. The O.R. was already booked for my biopsy at 1:00 that afternoon and he was there to tell me what would be done. When I questioned his haste to cut me open, he told me there was no time to waste. "Hmmm… not going to be an infection," I thought. As I rose from the bed, he asked where I thought I was going and my response, "Home" was not to his liking. No one was cutting me open until I had a chance to think more clearly and hell, maybe even get a second opinion. Maybe I would wake up from this nightmare and it would all be just that — a bad dream and there would never be any cutting.

When I reached for my jeans and began removing my hospital gown, "Dr. Slice-em and Dice-em" informed me I could not leave. His face indicated the seriousness of his words. Undeterred,

I continued getting dressed amidst his demands that I sign a "discharge against medical advisement form" before they would let me leave. "Bring me a pen. I'll sign. I'm leaving."

Alone in the ER parking lot, I thought, "Could this be true? Could I really have cancer?" My hands shook noticeably, so much so I had difficulty putting the key into the ignition. Thousands of questions flooded my brain before I could drive away. What kind of cancer? Should I have stayed for the biopsy? Why didn't I ask more questions? How will I tell my family? What effect will this have on them? Unbridled, the mind will bolt from logical thought. And no matter how hard I tried to rein in the terror, I could not. And I was alone with no one to help hold the runaway mind at bay.

I do not know how I managed to drive myself home any more than I knew how I got to the hospital the night before. All I knew in that moment was that my life was about to change, dramatically, though I could not imagine how dramatically.

CHAPTER 2

S.O.S. THE SECOND OPINION SYNDROME

That the human mind is capable of experiencing so many feelings at one time is hard to fathom. Yet, one has only to be diagnosed with cancer to know how possible this is. Fear, immobility, denial, indecision, frustration anger, anxiety, dysfunction, humor, stress, resolve, loneliness. Did I overlook any?

Fear

The thought of seeking a second opinion was frightening. Different faces, new emotions. It was a double-edged sword. Do I want to go through more tests to find out the original diagnosis was right? And then what? Where do I go? How do I proceed?

Immobility

There is nothing in life that can prepare you for this—no teacher's manual with the answers in the back, no Cliff Notes to explain the plot, the characters and the outcome. And worse, did I want to know the answers? Should I ignore the first diagnosis? After all, I had gone to a second-rate hospital emergency room with less than competent doctors who were not all oncologists and who probably had to fill their monthly surgical quotas. They could be wrong. Right? Did I want to know how incompetent they were? It might very well be just an infection or even indigestion.

Denial

And what if a second opinion confirmed the first? Should I go for a third opinion or a fourth, *ad infinitum*, until I was convinced or grew too weary to fight the reality? Already my energy levels were being sapped and I had not even chosen a course of action.

Indecision

When is enough enough?

Frustration

Rational thinking eventually took over and I sought the opinion of my primary care physician, Kenneth Fishberger, who is an excellent diagnostician. He is caring, yet methodical. It would not be unusual to wait for 2-3 hours (with an appointment) to see him because he took his time with each of his patients. He has an edgy sense of humor, yet he leaves no stone unturned. And so it was that I went for more tests — MRI's, PET scans and CT scans — the alphabet soup of cancer diagnostics. When the results were in I returned to his office and I knew immediately from his face that the news was not good. He put his arm on my shoulder and said, "Jim, you need to go for a biopsy." I could feel my knees give way yet, oddly enough all I could think of in that moment was my grandchildren and not being able to see them grow up — nothing like jumping to the worst possible conclusion — and so he took over, made the appointment for the surgery leaving me to consider how I was going to proceed.

Anxiety and Loneliness

Until this point, I had told no one what I had been going through for the last ten days, opting to weather this alone rather than put anyone through unnecessary worry. I mean if it were nothing more than indigestion or an infection I could take some antacids or antibiotics and be done with this and no one would be the wiser.

Dysfunction

I must note how quickly my brain traveled from abject despair to unrealistic optimism. The emotional roller coaster had been set in motion.

It is said that timing is everything. And in this case it certainly was. The Christmas holidays were fast approaching. It was already mid-December and I did not want to put a damper on anyone's holiday spirit. One should not share one's angst, at least not yet. I would have sucked it up and dealt with it on my own but for the word biopsy being stamped on my brain in 24 point New Times Roman. Now, I had to break my code of silence and share this burden, which was growing heavier by the day. Besides, I needed a ride to the hospital and back on the day of the surgery.

Humor, *albeit* Gallows Humor

That job fell to Nancy, about whom I will write much more later. She always had been my support, my rock, and my conscience at times. She is the clear thinker when my mind begins to shut down and my brain suffers from acute constipation. We had been together for nineteen years at that time and it would have been impossible to keep this from her any longer. How I was able to for ten days, I'll never know. Must have been her preoccupation with holiday preparations that jammed her radar. For many who are diagnosed with cancer, their partners are there from the get-go and the breaking of this kind of news falls to the doctor. But for those of us who are single the onus falls squarely on us to tell a loved one. I thought this would be the hardest thing I would have to do. What did I know? I can remember sitting her down at the kitchen table and making her promise not to be angry with me for what I was about to say. Of course, the look on her face belied her confusion and rapidly growing concern. There followed the disbelief, the fear and then she shifted to her usual, "Okay. So where do we go from here?" mode. Unlike myself, who'd opt any day to think and think and think, instead of act, she was not one to sit for too long when confronted with a situation that demanded immediate attention. She is a problem solver, *par excellence*. Since the wheels were already in motion for the biopsy, that became the obvious next step. Her take charge attitude did not, however, successfully mask her saddening eyes and her face which was trying to smile.

And then the wait.

So much of fighting cancer is the waiting — waiting for an appointment, waiting for a doctor who is backed up with his appointments and running late, and the worst, waiting for test results to come back which will determine your future course of action — hell, your entire future. Plain and simple.

Stress.

The biopsy done, lymph nodes removed from my right armpit, we waited nearly a week for the results, a week of eternity.

And there we were again, perched at the kitchen table, awaiting the phone call. Locked into a deadly silence, and lack of eye contact. Each too afraid to speak or look in the other's eyes lest the dam burst sending a flood of emotions to overwhelm us both.

One of us, at least, had to maintain a clear head to hear what the doctor had to say and physically be able to write down what the next steps would be.

And then the phone rang, shattering the silence. Of course, there was the dramatic hesitation, one you'd likely see in a hokey, three hanky movie, and the furtive eye contact before picking up the phone and stop its incessant ringing.

CHAPTER 3

NHL

NHL? What the hell is that? National Hockey League? Why was he talking sports and not the results of my biopsy? Oh, I see. The biopsy showed cancer in my lymph nodes. I had non-Hodgkins Lymphoma — NHL — small B cell, indolent, follicular lymphoma. Whoa! Way too many words to process at one time. All I really heard clearly was "cancer" followed by the Charles Schultz adult-speak, "waa, waa waa, waa".

The Big C, huh? Talk about slap shots!

I repeated the doctor's words aloud — one, so that Nancy could hear them in the same time-space continuum that I was hearing them and two, so that I wouldn't have to repeat them to her after I hung up. Upon hearing the word cancer, she rose from the table and went swiftly into the other room. This would be the first of only two times she left my side unable to handle what she had heard or would see. I could hear her muffled crying from the living room as I concluded the conversation with the doctor. I must admit that all the while I was speaking with him and Nancy was in the other room, I had remained calm, clear-headed. My heart rate never rose, or at least I don't think it did. But in that moment, when we had to look into each other's faces, make real eye contact, everything changed. Her tear-streaked face, her eyes red and swollen and her quivering lower lip were the outward manifestations of what was roiling inside of me, banging at my insides, screaming to be let out.

It was real now. It was palpable. It was cancer. And it would become part of our lives. It would move in with us as an unwelcomed guest. It would take up residence in our present moments and haunt our subconscious. Somehow, at that moment, I vowed to allow it to be only part of our lives, of my life and not be my life.

Resolve

And so we held on to each other, as we would do many, many, more times, and all that was begging to be let out from inside of me came rushing forth. And we cried.

Without an oar to steer the shaky boat in the right direction and stop it from going around in circles, I again turned to to my internist for guidance. Sensing my helplessness he made a call to a friend and colleague of his — an oncologist — and secured for me an appointment after the holidays.

But the larger and more immediate problem now was how to tell the rest of my family - my sisters and their families, Nancy's children, and of course, my own children.

Cancer was about to become a family disease.

CHAPTER 4

A Theater of the Absurd Picnic

Pre-cancer life for me was about order — putting my toys away as child, making sure my clothes were neatly tucked into the dresser drawer. I learned early on how to order the priorities others had set for me. Whatever the case, it brought peace and harmony. I avoided confrontation, conflict and sometimes even having to think for myself. Once my priorities were set, my life would follow suit. Choices and decisions about what to do, where to go, what shirt to buy, who to marry, what job to take, became effortless. I wanted to hitchhike around Europe for eleven weeks and I did. I became a teacher instead of a dentist because the schooling was shorter, easier and I would make money faster, although I realized later it would not be nearly as lucrative. I wanted a family, so I got married.

Life was much simpler pre-cancer. It was like going on a picnic with all the trappings for a wonderful day. I took time and care filling the picnic hamper with all the goodies and found an idyllic spot in nature. The blanket was spread, the plates, forks and knives, the spoons, glasses and napkins arranged neatly in their proper places. From out the hamper came the chicken, the potato salad and the wine and I settled in comfortably to spend a leisurely day enjoying the fruits of the preparations. You get the idea.

Then, the diagnosis.

As if some invisible force picked up the four corners of the blanket and tossed the carefully planned and laid out picnic high into the air, nothing ended up where it was, where it was supposed to be. Plates were scattered here and there. Some were still whole; some were chipped and others lay in fragments and shards on the ground. Glasses, forks, spoons and knives were scattered, some lost. Napkins whirled and fluttered on the invisible air current. But nothing would be the same anymore. Nothing was where it should be. I tried to reset the blanket, restoring the picnic items to their paper place. But that proved impossible.

It was time to try to make sense of a life that had been turned upside down. Restore order. Re-prioritize things. Do I keep the chipped and broken plates, glueing them back together though the cracks would always be visual reminders of what life used to be. Or do I discard them. Do I need all the "fixins" I carried with me to this picnic or could I throw some them away, lightening the burden, making travel easier?

In the end, I carefully put back what still retained its meaning and importance, leaving behind what was unfixable and insignificant. I would spend the next part of my life trying to understand what had happened and trying to regain order in the face of great uncertainty. I am still working on that.

And so it was with confusion and fear, I had to tell my family and face the thousands of questions to which I had no answers.

Thought For The Day

I find television very educating. Every time someone turns
on the set, I go into the other room and read a book.

Mark Twain

CHAPTER 5

TELLING THE FAMILY

During a period of the next five years I came to learn many things. But of major significance is that I found myself trying to protect others from this disease, to shelter loved ones from what I was going to have to face. I cared more about their feelings than my own. Maybe I was avoiding having to deal with it all.

Holidays have always been difficult. The nuclear family unit, battered by divorces and new relationships and blended families made the logistics of telling the family — families — stressful especially during the fast approaching holidays.

The various factions of family were gathered and in time everyone was told after Christmas, including a flight to Florida to tell my daughter, Jamie. Things such as this should not be told over the phone and I wanted to be there as a shock absorber for her if needed.

Family reactions had little in common. Some were shocked and expressed their shock and fear as questions and concerns; others were silent, not knowing what to say. In fact, I found that most people did not know what to say or offered platitudes such as, "You look great. If you hadn't told me, I would never have known." To wit, I often replied, "Come crawl inside my body and see just how 'not great' I am". And still others let the tears flow down their cheeks in mute response to it all. I have learned to judge people only by their intentions and not by their words or lack thereof. All the responses were of good intent, regardless of how well or not-so-well they were expressed.

What followed was three years of chemo and scans. Relapses and protocol changes. Nothing was working. After each relapse the pain grew worse and the cancer undeterred, kept spreading. Several hospitalizations and near-death experiences re-echoed that what I was doing was not working. Difficult choices had to be made. "If you always do what you've always done, you'll always get what you always got." Ultimately, the decision was made to go to Memorial Sloan-Kettering in New York City to explore the possibilities of a stem cell transplant. In May, I met with the head of the transplant department and I was approved to move forward with the transplant. That summer, I would receive radiation treatments for 7 weeks, 5 days a week to prepare my body for what was to come. Though it took several months, a donor was found through the Bone Marrow Donor Registry. No one in my family was a match.

On January 15 of 2009, I met with the stem cell transplant team and a "definite" admission date of January 28 was established. Note the word definite is in quotes. As I came to learn, nothing in the world of cancer is definite. And relying on "definiteness" is the hobgoblin of foolish minds. Prior to admission I would have to go through a series of pre-treatment tests, some of which I had today. Long story very short, the donor is ready, willing and able and the stem cells will be harvested on February 2 or 3. On February 5, I will get the actual transplant after a week of high dose chemo and radiation and anti-rejection drugs. Looking forward to getting started and, of course, finishing successfully.

January 19. This was a difficult day in that it was long, stressful and debilitating —four pre-transplant tests. The weather did not cooperate either, complicating the day's travels. The loss of my gloves and glasses, by day's end, put the icing on the cake. What kept me going was the support of family and friends and having Nancy by my side. The caregivers, the unspoken heroes, remain in the shadows, offstage so to speak, waiting to make their entrance on cue as needed.

Thought For The Day

Be responsible for the energy you bring to others.

January 22. Flexibility. And so begins the first of many lessons to be learned — patience and flexibility. My admission date has been moved from next Wednesday, January 28 to somewhere closer to February 11. To the best of my knowledge, the postponement is due to having to have two teeth pulled today. They might cause a problem for my recuperation from the chemo and radiation and any infection might be fatal without an immune system to fight it. Another reason is that my donor would not be available for harvesting his/her stem cells until February 2 or 3. Without those there can be no transplant. It has been a busy day filled with phone calls and schedule changes. Energy levels rapidly depleting. However, despite the delays and disappointments, the power of prayer and support has kept me going. In particular I must mention the healing shawl that a former student, Rev. Keith Spencer's congregation made for me. It arrived today, touching me deeply.

Thought For The Day

Things happen. They don't ask first.
They don't need your permission.

February 4. Yesterday, I completed my final round of pre-transplant tests and the results of prior tests have come back 'normal'. With that good news, I was given another "definite" (there's that word again) admission date. One week from today, February 11, I will begin the next leg of this journey perhaps the most risk/reward part of it, to be sure. In a nutshell, for those of you curious enough to wonder, I will get 5 days of TBI — total body irradiation. What will follow will be a day of much needed rest, so I'm told. The donor's stem cells which will have been harvested by then, will be implanted sometime during the third week of February. The first hundred days will be the most critical in terms of the stem cells taking root and rebuilding my immune system.

Thought For The Day

The greatest good you can do for another is not just to
share your riches, but to reveal them to his own.

Benjamin Disraeli

February 10. Well, the time has come at last. I am both anxious and excited that this is finally going to start. Add nervous to the list of emotions. This is normal. But when it is happening to you, it feels anything but normal. People have been so kind, regaling me with stories of friends who have had stem cell transplants and have survived and thrived for five, seven, even ten years. I'm certainly hoping for longer, but this is certainly encouraging. The technology so many years ago was far from what it is today. New breakthroughs in stem cell research work only to my advantage, making me glad I did not get sick ten or twenty years ago. And so I go into tomorrow with a very positive outlook. Responses to my posts and your emails and cards bolster my strength. Harness all the energy sent my way, and I am ready to hit the ground running.

This past weekend Nancy presented me with the finished product — a magnificent, handmade quilt that she gave me for Christmas as a work-in-progress. It is a special reminder that I am not alone. I say these things to remind me and anyone whose life has been touched by cancer, that these gestures, whether great or small, are part of the healing process. They charge us with an energy to keep fighting and at the very least, put a smile on our face.

I am already looking forward to the spring and the start of the golf season. Hopefully, after this winter's hiatus I will have forgotten all of my bad habits and only the good will remain, however few they are.

PART II

THE BLOG ENTRIES

What follows in Part 2 is a series of entries from my Caring Bridge Blog. These entries are divided into two sections: one - pre-transplant (the days labelled T-) and two - post transplant (T+). It is during this time that I met some of the most interesting people whose stories and faces are with me today. Their journeys forced me to look at my own more carefully and realize there are so many people whose struggles are far more difficult than my own.

"It's important that everyone knows
that I'm so much more than the bad things that happen to me."

Jane Marczewski
Nightbirde

CHAPTER 6

HURRY UP AND WAIT

February 12. And so it begins. As with many things, the travel was not all that smooth yesterday. Delays in getting into my room kept Nancy and me waiting for over seven hours and I was finally moved from a ward-like area into the first available room on the transplant floor at about 10:00 PM. It is small, but it is private and far better for me health-wise to be here. I have queued myself to getting into a larger room when one becomes available. For those of you who are thinking dirty thoughts about queuing myself, and you know who you are, it simply means I've put my name on a list and I'm in line (the queue) to be "moving on up" to better accommodations.

I know the old joke about a sailor wanting a girl in every port or a little port in every girl, but now I have my own port and a very decorative one to say the least. It is not the under the skin kind but rather is outside my chest and I have three leads that go into my jugular vein. These leads look like they've been beaded so either I teleported to Jamaica and had what remains of my chest hair braided or I can now get a job as a pole dancer at some over 60 dance club as I have what can pass for a tassel on my right pectoral muscle — neither of which is a pretty image.

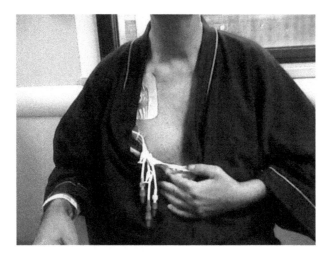

They started my chemo regimen this morning and so far so good. This may be a bit premature as most of the side effects won't kick in for a while and today is only the first infusion. In Sloan-Kettering-speak it is Day T-6. In layman's terms that is six days before transplant. So I am making myself as comfortable as possible in my little bubble. The nursing staff has been excellent, caring and attentive. They are personable and friendly and have great senses of humor. I am most grateful for that.

Thought For The Day

Being happy doesn't mean everything is perfect. It means you've decided to look beyond the imperfections.

February 14. Happy Valentine's Day. Here it is Day T-4, four days to go until the transplant. I have grown accustomed to the short leash I'm on. I know I ended the sentence with a preposition, but "I've grown accustomed to the short leash on which I am" sounds way too pedantic and stodgy. But I digress. My IV pole has no less than 6 or 7 drip bags hanging from it at any given time. I have to plug and unplug myself whenever I move more than a couple of feet. But seeing as I haven't been moved to a larger room yet, I can cover most of my living space with some creative maneuvers. Showering, however, presents a real challenge of getting under the shower head without dragging my now constant, skinny companion, my IV pole, with me. Right now there are no larger rooms available and I don't know if one will become available any time soon. But I can hope. The sad thing is that if I change rooms I won't have the same nurses and they have been truly kind and supportive.

Nancy just left after a wonderful visit this afternoon. It made my V-Day extra special having her here. My sister also visited this AM and I was grateful for her company as well. It is good to laugh heartily and often. The strange thing is that I don't mind being by myself on occasion because I know I can always find company. But when I'm forced into being alone, with no chance of parole, "alonenesss" turns to loneliness. Visits from family and friends are the most potent medicine.

Thought For The Day

—∞∞∞—

To love someone is to see him as God intended him.

Fyodor Dostoyevsky

FEBRUARY 15. T-3

It is Sunday and the transplant is on schedule for Wednesday. After the last four days of high-dose chemo (with the last one tomorrow) they have started me on the anti-rejection drugs, the side effects of which should not be discussed in public. But as I look at it, I am one day closer to the transplant and one day closer to being cured. Once Wednesday comes (called Day 0) we start counting forward as in T+1 and so on, until the first 100 days have passed. That is the most critical time, for it is then that I could develop an infection or the donor's stem cells might not graft properly and I'll be back to square one. I am fortunate that my donor is a 10 point match for me i.e. his/her stem cells won't reject my body but I am only a 9 point match for my donor which means my body might not accept them, hence the anti-rejection drugs.

Many have asked if I know my donor. I do not. According to the Bone Marrow Donor Registry, we will remain anonymous to each other for a year. If after that time he/she wants to have his identity revealed, then we can contact each other. What a wonderful thing it would be for me to thank this person for this gift. I get goosebumps just thinking of the possibility of that moment. I have been warned that many donors wish to maintain their anonymity. My friend Janet, a donor herself, explained her reason for remaining anonymous was simple. "It is a gift," she said, "and I want no credit or recognition." Still other donors do not want the relationship if things do not go well. Whatever the reason there is little else I can think of that demonstrates the generosity of spirit of all donors who have given to others, strangers in many cases, a second chance at life.

As a side bar, I'm getting fat, as difficult as that may be to believe. Much is due to the chocolate covered cherries from my sister and the Godiva chocolates from Nancy. I am sharing the "C.C.C" with the nursing staff because they are so wonderful, but not so wonderful as to merit the Godivas. They are all mine!

Thought For The Day

Be kinder than necessary, for everyone you meet is fighting some kind of battle.

CHAPTER 7

BEST LAID PLANS AND THEN SOME

Instead of today being T-2 it is now T-1. Yes, they have moved he transplant up to tomorrow, not Wednesday! I will be getting total body irradiation in the morning and then the transplant later in the day. All of this is good news especially after yesterday and most of today the side effects of the anti-rejection drugs were devastating. Not only did I have them all, but I had them in their most severe form. I am feeling better now— I always marvel at the human body and how much it is able to withstand and how it is able to recuperate. Perhaps I am feeling better because of the nine bags of medications and chemo hanging from my IV pole or the good news that tomorrow will be Day Zero. Apparently the donor's stem cells took an earlier flight than expected and wanted to get settled in prior to the original arrival time.

Strike up the band. Let the party in my bone marrow begin.

Of special note here is another one of those gifts you receive from a person you admire greatly and which comes without warning. Anthony Griffin, a former student of mine and now close friend, is teaching all the classes I taught when I retired. Anthony took one of the projects I loved doing with my students and tweaked it to make it his own. It is called the Quilt Project. Simply, the quilt project uses student writing as the patches of the quilt bordered by a colorful, traditional pattern. The students dedicated the quilt to me and named it "How to Make the World a Better Place".

It was gratifying to know I had passed this project on to him and he was now returning the gift to me tenfold. Cancer touches so many lives, not just the patients' or caregivers'. The faces of his students in the photos he sent, beamed with pride. Their caring and concern for me was obvious.

Thought For The Day

---∞∞∞---

Life isn't about waiting for the storm to pass. It is about learning to dance in the rain.

CHAPTER 8

THE DAY OF RECKONING — DAY ZERO

This is the day I have been waiting for since last May when I first met with the oncologists at Sloan. From this day forward I will count in positive integers until Day+100 is but a fading memory. Today's itinerary includes Total Body Irradiation (TBI) in the morning and then the actual transplant sometime in the late afternoon. Both anxious and excited about today, I could not fall back asleep after the morning blood draws and weigh-in at 4:00 AM. To pass the time, I listened to the iPod my daughter Jamie, Mykayla and Ryan gave me for Christmas. The play selection was set to random. Ironically, the first song to play was Etta James' "At Last"! But even more incredible is what followed: "Hooked on a Feeling", "Let's Get this Party Started" and as I thought about Nancy's visit today, "Pretty Woman" started to play. A friend once told me that there is no such thing as coincidence. It is only God's way of remaining anonymous. Can't ask for a better wing man than God and so I will take all that as a good omen.

The TBI went very smoothly, a walk in the park in comparison to what I have already been through. No side effects whatsoever. I was told before the TBI began that 50% of the people puke, and though I had just eaten breakfast, no scrambled eggs found their way to the floor.

At a few minutes after 4:00 PM EST the stem cells entered the building and just a bit later, at 4:34 PM I was "wired" so to speak.

The hook ups had been made, the valves opened and my new life's blood began to flow. February 17th is now my new birthday, in case you were thinking of buying me a gift or baking me a cake.

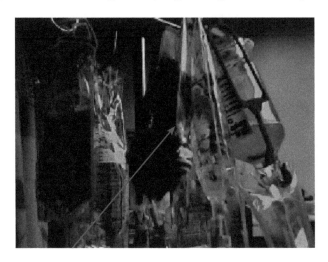

I was glad Nancy was there to witness this miracle of generosity which we discovered was neither painless nor convenient. The harvesting of the stem cells took two days, and only after the donor had received several weeks of injections to stimulate his/her stem cell growth insuring the transplant would be viable and successful.

A little pouch measuring about 8"x10", emptied what could have passed for a rich marinara sauce (maybe the donor is Italian!) into my veins where the stem cells would find their way to my bone marrow, each with its own microscopic GPS, and reproduce, giving me a new blood type, a new immune system, a new DNA and hopefully a new, long and healthy life.

With the transplant completed, I thought it was safe to exhale.

Not.

The rigors set in and my body began to shake uncontrollably. I thought then that my life would end with a shiver and not a bang. Or that my body was rejecting the stem cells and all this had been for naught. Once again the nursing staff seized the moment, not only administering Demerol to stop the shakes, but more importantly the kindness in their faces told me I would be all right. They held my hand and comforted me and alleviated my fears and I drifted off into sleep.

Thought For The Day

───⬳⬲⬲⬳───

When God takes something from your grasp, He's
not punishing you, but merely opening your hands to
receive something better.

CHAPTER 9

T+1 AND T+2

Suffice it to say that those stem cells threw one helluva party and unfortunately, the host — me — paid handsomely for it. It was not one of my better days to say the least. All kinds of medical complications arose for which the medical profession has all kinds of cures, which cause other complications for which there are all kinds of cures etc, *ad nauseam*. Every cancer patient and caregiver knows this and my experiences yesterday were by no means unique. By 9 PM most of the complications had been brought under control and the evening was capped off by some good news — I was next in the queue to move into a bigger room. Fortunately, my sister Laurie was there to help me pack my things and within an hour I was in my new digs. I have a view of York Avenue, with a glimpse of the 59th Street Bridge, but more significantly, I can see the sky and feel the sun beating through the window. For a week, I had seen nothing but the grey side of another wing of the hospital with no light or sky in sight. Once again I am reminded how important the little things are.

This morning, with the window shade up and the sun beating down into my room, I enjoyed breakfast, with no migraine headache or nausea to interfere with the simple beauty of it all. However, it seems the stem cell party, which wreaked havoc on the host was about to continue. The invited guests were the Platelet family. Hopefully they will bring decorum to the revelers and calm them down. My only fear is that their kissing cousins, the Hemoglobins, are due to arrive in the next few days. And you know how undependable they can be. So we shall see who prevails. Meanwhile, the Lasix, you know them, the next door neighbors, have made bathroom travel quite frequent.

Obviously, I am feeling much better today. I won't say 'normal' for I have forgotten what normal feels like, and I fear the wicked backlash I might incur, but I'm most grateful for being, at the minimum, functional.

Thought For The Day

———◦∞∞◦———

So, if you feel a smile begin, don't leave it undetected.
Let's start an epidemic quick and get the whole world
infected.

Russel H. Conwell

Chapter 10

Day T+3

Day T+2 passed relatively uneventfully, other than a brief visit from the Platelets and another wanging migraine-like headache, which seems to have medical science baffled as to their recurrence. My theory, though I am not doctor, nor do I play one on TV, is that they got caught up in their partying and went on a feeding frenzy on the residual Jack Daniels left in my system from last season in Florida. It was enough to throw their young innocent cell souls into a tailspin, leaving my body to clean up the mess. Tsk…Tsk…

My sister Susan called today. Whenever she calls, she says, "You're never feeling well when I call." I told her, "So, stop calling then." She is visiting tomorrow which should break the chain of her bad luck phone calls.

I have discovered my neighbors, the Lasix, own and operate Lasix Airlines and they have been kind enough to give me double frequent pee-er miles. I now have logged enough of those miles to pee just about anywhere in the world!

Day T+4

Despite the wonderful visit from my sister yesterday, today was a difficult day. The migraines persist and the only thing that seems to subdue them is Imitrex, a drug that caused my pulse rate to double the first time it was administered. However, today's covering physician came up with the perfect solution, one which I had suggested several days before… even though I'm still not a doctor… "She said drink coffee or have a Coke. You're suffering from caffeine withdrawal." True, the coffee here is horrible so I stopped drinking it several days ago. So no more migraines or hard drugs. It's good ole 7-11 high octane for me.

Today I look forward to Nancy's visit. I miss her so much — her laugh, her dancing blue eyes, her infinite kindness. She doesn't know yet but during today's non-conjugal visit, she gets to rub Eucerin cream all over my body, twice. Doctor's orders — honestly! There are perks to having dry skin from all the chemo.

Thought For The Day

When you reach the end of your rope,
tie knot in it and hang on.

Thomas Jefferson

Chapter 11

Day T+5

Happy to report that now that I am doing Coke, the headaches have subsided. I even choked down a cup of Sloan coffee for extra good measure. Not quite the same as a Starbuck's Mocha Latte. If I could just break out of my room and run down to the local 7-11, I would. But, the door to my room is heavily barricaded by nasty-looking, burly guards wielding hefty-looking syringes. I cannot help but wonder just what is in coffee that is stronger than morphine or cocaine and why are so many of us addicted to it.

Other than another visit from the Platelets last night to help stop any bleeding, I am handling the side effects pretty well. I am at my most vulnerable now. Literally, I have no immune system and am susceptible even to the most minor infection. It will take another week and a half before my counts start to rise and I will be less at risk.

Despite my crackerjack detective work, my stem cells did not come from a donor in Minneapolis, MN. That is where the National Bone Marrow Donor Registry is located, and my day nurse, Sylvia — a gem with a kind and caring manner — confirmed that the stem cells or their pouch or both somehow go through MN before arriving at their final destination. The markings on the pouch were a red herring and so back to square one, Inspector Clouseau!

Today the Sunday brunch menu offers tomato basil soup, whole wheat pancakes in maple syrup butter and key lime pie. Not sure what the dinner specials are yet so I'll wait to place my 'room service' order. The nurse changed my bed linens from yesterday and gave me a fresh supply of towels. In some respects, life ain't too bad. Room and maid service included. It almost makes me forget why I'm here. Well, almost.

But in a world of tradeoffs the wonderful day I spent with Nan yesterday was well-worth the great sadness I felt when she had to leave. As she walked down the hall, turned right and disappeared from view, a great sadness set in. An over-abiding loneliness.

Thought For The Day

While we may not be able to control all that happens to us, we can control what happens inside of us.

Benjamin Franklin

CHAPTER 12

DAY T+6

My room is approximately a 20x20 space, in which are a cabinet a closet, a bookcase, a small computer shelf, my bed, a nightstand and an ominous panel of input and output valves. There is a bathroom off to the right of my bed, one which is functional at best. The window overlooking York Avenue which I mentioned earlier, is hermetically sealed, shutting out any germs or infectious bacteria as well as any sounds except for the strident chirp of an ambulance pulling up to the main entrance of the hospital.

The door to my room has a small window with a pull down shade. Outside noise can be heard but there is little other than the occasional murmurs of visitors or the soft sounds of the staff as they pad up and down the hallway ministering to the sick. The snap of a non-latex glove against a wrist and a gentle rap on the door are the only harbingers of their arrival to take vitals and hang more bags on the IV poles — the constant companions of cancer patients. There is other noise from adjacent rooms — a chair being dragged across the floor, the muted beeping of IV pumps, the flushing of a toilet. These are the sounds of the living.

I am cut off from the world. It is lonely. It is claustrophobic. And at times it seems that all this will never come to an end. Last night as I was brushing my teeth I looked in the mirror at this old man, with grey hair and stubble on his face, and I got angry. I got angry because of what this disease has done to me in the last two years plus. I got angry for what has been taken from me and what it has left me with. I got angry because I cannot shave with a regular razor because if I cut myself I could bleed out. I got angry for not being able to spend time with loved ones or be in Florida right now. I got angry because the mass of tubes coming from my chest tangle with the electric cords which run the pumps that hum and whirr incessantly and insidiously beep in the middle of the night and cast ghastly green shadows on the walls and ceiling and interrupt sleep. I got angry because I cannot use the webcam to talk to and video conference with my daughters and grandchildren because it is "against hospital policy". I got angry at the cancer, not the world. I got angry because I could not scream at it and tell it to leave me alone.

I am better today. But I still cannot scream.

Thought For The Day

The power to believe in yourself is the
power to change fate.

CHAPTER 13

DAY T+7

Today I start the Neupogen shots which are designed to rebuild my immune system by stimulating cell growth — in my case, my donor cells. I have had Neupogen shots in the past and they are painful to get, cause severe bone and joint pain and gave me migraine headaches for a week. Hmmm, this is beginning to sound all too familiar. If I drink any more caffeine they will have to scrape me off the ceiling, not too many other places to escape in my room. However, when I spoke to the doctor about trying to fend off these headaches, he said he would check my white cell count to see if they were necessary. One thing I have learned is to ask questions and never just accept the *status quo*. And to keep asking questions or have a patient advocate with you to ask questions. Only moments ago I found out based on the number of cells donated, I won't have to have the shots. Don't ask me who counted them all, but there were over 6.5 million stem cells in the "harvest". Usually 5 million is the sought after baseline, so I am well into the plus column. Imagine counting and at 6.4 million you are distracted and have to start all over again. One, two, three.....but I digress. No wonder those pesky little guys were wreaking havoc the first few days. Hopefully, most of them have settled into their new home and taken up residence in my bone marrow, where they will begin to replicate themselves as stems cells are wont to do. Go stem cells! Go stem cells!

Thought For The Day

Never hire a color blind electrician.

CHAPTER 14

DAY T +8

Week three. Hard to believe that a week ago I received the transplant and those 6.5 million puppies are doing their thing hopefully. I will find out just how well they are faring when I get my counts today. And speaking of counts:

Over the last two weeks I have learned that it is the simple things that count and very often those are the things we most take for granted.

For example:

Eating a home cooked meal, chemo taste buds notwithstanding
Peeing into a toilet rather than into a portable urinal
Sleeping in a queen size bed, preferably with someone, rather than in a single bed whose mattress grunts and groans and re-inflates to adjust with my every movement
Walking untethered to an IV pole
Taking a shower untethered to the above
Touching someone not through rubber gloves or a glass window, but rather skin to skin
Kissing lips, touching cheeks, hugging
Watching HD TV on a flat screen
Watching the Golf Channel on any TV
Hugging a granddaughter up close and personal
Hearing her giggle, smelling her skin

Drinking real coffee, smelling its rich aroma
Playing golf with good friends
Walking in the sunshine and feeling the sun's warmth on my skin

Well, you get the idea.

I know this will sound crazy, even a bit trite, but I honestly believe that I have made it this far and other than the headaches and a few bad days, I have handled the side-effects of the transplant fairly well, primarily because of the prayers and positive energy sent my way. The jokes and funny emails have insulated me from descending into dark thoughts and worst case scenarios. The doctors say that I am doing well and that I am in better shape at this point than many of the other patients on this floor. On days T+12 - T+14 my counts should increase and that will be the first measure of how well the transplant has succeeded.

Thought For The Day

⸺⧉⸺

Never go to a doctor whose office plants have died.

Erma Bombeck

Day T+ 9

Add to yesterday's list of things taken for granted:

A full night's uninterrupted sleep
Being able to sneeze without causing a bloody nose
Being able to cough without setting off multiple IV pumps and monitors
Being as strong as possible going into this

Yesterday, the housekeeping person told me (although she probably should not have) about a young man down the hall from me, 27 years old, married. His wife had just had their first child and he had leukemia. He is from upstate NY and his wife cannot visit him because of the recent birth; his mother has six other children and the round trip from Albany, would take her most of the day so she can visit only occasionally. He is very, very sick and the radiation he has been given is significantly more than I received. He is suffering from radiation burns so much so that his skin is peeling off making him that much more susceptible to infection. The pain meds they are administering make him so groggy that he cannot stay awake, let alone advocate for himself.

Again I am reminded that without a support system this disease is so difficult to battle. With no one to advocate for you, you are more alone than ever. I am grateful for the support from family which makes sure things are all right, bring me home cooked meals, do my laundry and love me.

In other news, yesterday I spoke with Dr. Perales. He felt all was going well and because of the high concentration of stem cells, the chances of success are 98%. As one can imagine, this brought a big smile. Nothing is 100% but as far as odds go, I like those. Because I am not going to get the Neupogen shot to stimulate cell growth, my counts will not start to rise until T+16 - T+18 instead of T+12 - T+14. I will gladly wait those extra days just to avoid the headaches.

The Platelets are due to arrive at any moment, as are their distant cousins, the Hemoglobins. Counts were way down this morning, which is normal, *albeit* a little scary. But this is standard protocol so I have been told. So move over stem cells. You are going to have to share a room.

Thought For The Day

Blessed is he who has learned to laugh at himself for he
shall never cease to be amused.

John Boswell

CHAPTER 15

DAY T+10

There was a jockeying for position yesterday at the Bone Marrowdrome. Counts were down so the Platelets and the Hemoglobins were brought in to line up against the home town Stem Cell team. Because they were heavily outnumbered, the P's and H's brought in a ringer — the Pre-Meds — and knocked the host on his proverbial butt. I spent a good part of the day vegging out and did not accomplish much. I was hoping to clean out the garage, paint the living room and caulk the master bath! But those will have to wait. In my dreams I was able to clean my golf clubs though.

Looking forward to this afternoon and another special home-cooked dinner courtesy of Meals on Wheels of Bluepoint. And on Saturday, the arrival of the Chocolate Chip Cookie Wagon of Patchogue, delivered with loving care by my daughter, Kristen, and her fiancé, Mike.

There are many things to look forward to in my life. But each has to be considered in small steps, one day at a time. Each day that passes is one less I have to experience again and one day closer to T+100 I get.

And today, I get to take a "hands-free" shower unencumbered by any tubes or wires. Whoopee! And my port dressing will be changed. Such is the kind of room service they offer here.

In other good news, today my counts are up from yesterday. Amazing what a transfusion or two will do. I am still trying to get them to transfuse me with some Jack Daniels; but I'm not having much luck on that front.

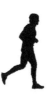

Thought For The Day

Some people walk in the rain. Others just get wet.

Roger Miller

CHAPTER 16

DAY T+11   THE GOOD, THE BAD AND THE UGLY.

The Good:

I can now get CBS! I had already applied to the hospital's methadone clinic for recovering Golf Addicts. But for now, no need.

My night nurse, Aya — An absolute angel of mercy. Smart, efficient, caring, considerate and funny.

The Bad:

The food. Enough said.

Elisabetta, the Urine Nazi. She comes to the room in the pre-dawn hours and demands my urine.

The Ugly:

Hair... the Final Frontier. Well, it has begun. All I had hoped against has come to fruition. Losing my hair is the definitive proof that I have been treated for cancer. It is the ultimate symbol of this disease. Well, not the ultimate, but I'm not going there. There were warning signs early on. The IV port in my arm when my first chemo was given in 2007. Walking though the infusion room and seeing all the other patients I realized I, too, was now a cancer patient. Seeing a woman getting chemo through a port in her chest. I now have my own port and am an official member of that 'elite' group. However, the IV in my arm and the port in my chest can be concealed under a long sleeved shirt. A bald head, though it can be hidden under a cap, is still a bald head and noticeable as such. And although it is now fashionable for men to shave their heads, this is no fashion statement. This is more like a badge, a Distinguished Medal of Survival, so to speak. Am I worried about what I'm going to look like? I won't lie. Sure, a little. Do I care? Not really. I'd rather be bald and alive than have a full head of hair and be sick. I've already done the healthy hair/sick body schtick. So I will wear my badge proudly.

It will probably freak some people out, but it will still be me under that shiny pate. I join the ranks of my future son-in-law and brother-in-law. I'm guessing that I will look more like the illegitimate lovechild of Gandhi and Nosferatu. I'm girding myself for the onslaught of jokes. Bring 'em!

Thought For The Day

⸺⋙⋘⸺

Anyone seeing the family resemblance?

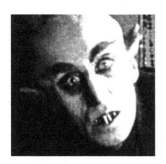 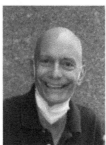 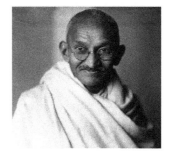

CHAPTER 17

DAY T+12

My counts are slowly rising. This is a good thing. Without the Neupogen shot it was expected to take longer. This week will be the telling week to see how well the stem cells have taken root and how well my body is making a new immune system for itself.

The transplant team just left and to quote the attending, "I've graduated". They are taking me off some of the IV drip meds and allowing me to take them orally. This is a big step because one, I cannot be discharged with an IV pole— would make for really awkward tee shots— and two, if my body weren't tolerating the drug regimen it would mean that I would have to stay incarcerated until I could. I am getting closer to 'blowing dis joint'!

Today is going to be a tough one. With the impending storm and the forecast for upwards of a foot of snow across Long Island, Nancy is not going to visit. I certainly do not want her to get caught here if the storm starts earlier and worsens sooner. This is really the suckiest part of this ordeal.

Hair update: still here, but rapidly thinning. One of the transplant team jokingly told me, "Don't worry. It will come back — curly and red!" Not ready for a starring role in 'Annie' just yet. But I have heard that when the hair comes back it might return with different texture and color.

It has begun. I'm molting! My hair is shedding into my dinner. I found the pelt of a dead animal in the shower basin, only to realize it was a clump of my own hair. I summoned the nurse with the razor and hastened the inevitable. Hair today, gone tomorrow!

Thought For The Day

―――∞∞∞――――

Life is like an onion. You peel off one
layer at a time and sometimes you weep.

Carl Sandburg

CHAPTER 18

DAY T+13

Today I am almost thankful to be in the hospital without the responsibility of shoveling walkways and cleaning off the car or simply being outside. The streets below did not look particularly bad this AM but just minutes ago it started snowing heavily. It is pretty to look at from an 8th floor perspective but I am glad I don't have to go out into it.

I am down to only two meds via IV drip. The rest are taken orally. Today the nurse taught me how to use a syringe to draw the two meds that are liquid. They are not injected, but administered orally.

Many of you have asked to hear more about Elisabetta, the Urine Nazi. I have such perverse friends. In stature Elisabetta closely resembles Bebe Neuwirth's character, Lilith, on "Frasier" — tall, thin, ebony hair pulled back into a severe bun, pale features, sunken eyes and I am sure dark red/black goth-like lips hidden beneath her surgical mask. I truly believe she sports fishnets and stilettos under her scrubs and secretly wields an Indiana Jones whip when no one is watching. When she barged into the room, storm-trooper-like, she would demand my urine. More often than not, I would be asleep or knowing it was she, I would pretend to be asleep. Then she would check the bathroom, realize I had given at the office and I could hear the indignant click-clack of her heels signaling her departure and my return to sleep.

At 4 AM one particular morning Elisabetta came to draw blood. I believe she took fiendish delight in the hour. She drew blood, flushed the line and asked the proverbial question, "Do you haff any urine for me?" Disappointed, she click-clacked her way down the hall. About an hour later I felt an excruciating pain in my side each time I rolled over in bed. Fearing something was terribly wrong I went into the bathroom to check. From one of my lines, hung the empty flush syringe, which had been digging into my side. When I called for the nurse, Elisabetta arrived. "Do you haff urine for me now?"

"No," I said, "but is this supposed to be here?" lifting my shirt and pointing to the syringe. Of course, she went into denial. "I sought I took everting out. It vas dark." She removed the syringe and left somewhat sheepishly, her demeanor softened and she padded, not click-clacked, her way out of the room.

I never saw her again. But now and then I hear a muted page in the middle of the night, "Elisabetta, please indicate" — i.e. answer the page — so I know she is out there, lurking, demanding urine in the night from some other unsuspecting fool.

And now for other news. The transplant team was in this AM and I asked what I should be looking for in terms of my counts that will determine my release date. The answer was both thrilling and terrifying. I could be discharged as early as this weekend or the beginning of next week. This is terrifying, as up until now, all my needs have been met round the clock. Now, I will have to start taking care of myself and that, at first, is going to be a complicated process. The thrilling part is that I am being discharged almost three weeks earlier than expected. And that, in large measure, is due to all the prayers, positive energy and support I have been given. For patients, this is as potent a medicine as any given by the oncologists and nurses. The prayers brought me a rich harvest of stem cells. The positive energy facilitated my body's acceptance of the stem cells. And the good thoughts kept me insulated from what could have been severe and long lasting side effects.

The next leg of the journey would be played out at Hope Lodge, an American Cancer Society sponsored housing facility near Penn Station. Alas, probably no more colorful characters like Elisabetta at Hope Lodge, but as I would come to learn, the people I would meet here would be the real faces of cancer.

Thought For The Day

—∞∞—

Thousands of candles can be lighted from a single
candle and the life of the candle will not be shortened.
Happiness never decreases by being shared.

Buddha

PART III

CHAPTER 19

DAY T+16

My counts are still trying to stabilize. Some have. Some have not. Among the have-nots are the most important ones, which will determine my release date. They are still fluctuating. I was told that this is to be expected because I declined the Neupogen shot. In reality, the timing may work out for the best as presently there are no rooms at the inn — a.k.a. Hope Lodge — until Wednesday. If they give me the boot before then, I will be roaming the streets of NYC, masked, gloved and bald in an open-back hospital gown. And that won't be a pretty sight. So much of the difficulty in dealing with the disease is the scheduling and the timing. And seemingly even when everything is in place, nothing is definite and everything is subject to change. The mechanics of cancer. Laurie is coordinating the effort and it is a massive task. I have always struggled with not being able to do things for myself. However, there are times when I have had to surrender my stubborn independent streak and let others take over. Right now we are awaiting a definite discharge date and hopefully, Laurie will be able to finalize the schedule so that the hired home care people can be given definite shifts. I am looking forward to my "freedom" on so many levels. It is just around the corner. I must be patient. I must be patient. I must be patient.

Thought For The Day

One of the keys to happiness is a bad memory.

Rita Mae Brown

Day T+17

I am suffering from "spring-me" fever. Not only is the weather warming up and hopefully there will be no mid/late month snowstorms, but I am also itching to get out in the fresh air and walk unrestricted. It has been a long time in the "slammer". I am fortunate that this part of my treatment has been shorter than expected. I cannot imagine going another three weeks. I guess if I had to I would.

The transplant team just finished rounds and are zoning in on next week if my counts continue to rise. Whether I leave with the port in my chest or not is still in question. Part of me wants it out. It is inconvenient at best. The other part of me says if they are going to be drawing blood 2-3 times a week, do I want to become a human pin cushion? My veins are becoming less and less viable from all the sticks. They roll over or blow and the process must be repeated. Neither choice is 100%.

The good news is that Elisabetta will not be my home care nurse. For now that will be shared by my friends, sisters and children and of course, Nancy. I am relieved that there will not be any misplaced syringes.

Thought For The Day

It is better to be patient than become one.

Day T+18

From my 8th floor perch today looks to be glorious. The sun is shining brightly, not a cloud in the sky. People are walking the streets clad in light-weight clothing, un-gloved and un-scarved. They are moving at a normal if not casual pace unlike their hurried, quickened steps of earlier this week. The day shift nurses arrive in upbeat moods, singing Spring's praises. As my friend Elaine mentioned in her post, "What better season to be discharged than Spring, the time of re-birth. I came here as one person, a person with cancer. I was given a second shot at life via the generosity of another human being and my body is being reborn.

I am looking forward to spending time with family and friends in a much less restricted environment at Hope Lodge. Each step is closer to coming home and while the steps might be small ones, they are taking me in the right direction. There are so many patients on this floor who are not moving forward, not moving at all or backsliding. And that is sad. I am most fortunate.

And in honor of Spring's much anticipated arrival…

Thought For The Day

To plant a garden is to believe in tomorrow.

Chapter 20

Day T+19

Daylight savings in the hospital is not quite as wonderful as it is outside these walls. It means the loss of an hour's sleep for all of us, sure. But for those of you who were not awakened by Vampira at 4 AM to draw your blood, take your vitals, get you out of bed to get weighed; who were not awakened by IV pump alarms beeping every half hour; or an ambitious doctor doing early rounds and a nursing assistant who just had to take your vitals again, that loss of an hour's sleep is akin to losing your best friend. Days will be longer now and hopefully in 3-4-5 days, freer too.

Discussion with my oncologist today included getting a lower dose Neupogen shot than before to avoid severe headaches. Waiting for my counts to rise is, according to him, like watching paint dry. My counts were duly offended by the analogy. I am faced with the inevitability of getting the shot. He said he could wait another day before making a decision about the shot to see what the counts do on their own. Removal of the port is also in question. Ahhh… life in Limbo!

Thought For The Day

If you surrender completely to the moments as they pass, you live more richly those moments.

Anne Morrow Lindbergh

DAY T+20

Well, it looks like Thursday is V-S Day — Victory at Sloan. The day of liberation. My counts have risen sufficiently and barring any deviation tomorrow or Wednesday, "I'm outta here" as they say. To paraphrase Dr. Martin Luther King, "Free at last! Thank God Almighty, I'll be free at last". No more IV pole tagging along wherever I go. Wireless showers all the time. No more urine collection (Eat your heart out Elisabetta!) No more pump alarms. No more 4 AM wake up calls. No more Sloan Slop for meals. No more incarceration in my 20x20 cell. So many things to be free of and so many more to celebrate ahead of me. The scheduling of the port removal has not been determined, but that, like my many other restraints, might be a thing of the past. I'll be a pin cushion. At this point I don't much care. What price freedom?

I had a good home-cooked meal last night from Meals on Wheels of Bluepoint, and life is good. Still, I must remember one day at a time. I have 80 days to go before I am in the safe zone; but today's news is certainly a giant step in the right direction.

For the next two days I will be taking classes in exit strategies and life on "the outside". I am feeling much like what rehabbed prisoners feel on the day they are set free. I wonder if I will get a new suit and $50 in my pocket. Maybe that is only a movie myth, like the myth of marijuana to curtail the side effects of chemo or the ice cream party I was promised as a child to get me to the hospital for a tonsillectomy.

Thought For The Day

A smile is an inexpensive way to change your looks.

Charles Gordy

Day T+21

Today I'm being treated for termites. And I thought getting out of here would be as simple as packing my belongings and walking out the door. It seems there are so many procedures that have to be followed before one can be released. Tenting is one of them. After rounds this AM I thought I was good to go. No mention of any further treatments except one more immune system bolstering drug. Moments after the team left, a respiratory therapist entered the room and said he was here to tent me. I looked at him incredulously. No one on rounds had said anything about this. And so tent in hand, he began to put me into this vinyl cocoon. When I requested to speak with my doctor before this was done he left indignantly. To this day, I still do not know how patients who are not well-enough to advocate for themselves when family is not present manage to survive. Anyway, the procedure, as it turns out, is to prevent me from getting pneumonia. Great. Another thing to worry about. An hour later I was tented for 30 minutes breathing in this noxious medication. Sometimes the cure, I fear, is worse than the disease. I am now proud to say that I am termite, roach and mealy worm free and it is guaranteed for a month when perhaps I'll have to be tented again depending on any new infestation.

Tomorrow I am getting another transfusion of platelets, and although my platelet numbers are good, this, like the tenting in a vinyl sheath is prophylactic. No comments. I also learned that the transfusion is the precursor to removing the port, likely tomorrow. Another step closer.

Thought For The Day

———∞∞∞———

Life is the movie you see through your own eyes. It makes little difference what's happening out there. It's how you take it that counts.

Denis Waitley

CHAPTER 21

For the many who read yesterday's post and punned me back, you did not disappoint. You relieved much "tent-sion" and made me laugh and made me remember how important laughter is in the healing process.

Moments ago I found out that my port will be removed this evening or tomorrow morning in preparation for my departure. And today, on the eve of my discharge, one month to the day after being admitted, I started reflecting on heroism.

Many people think that cancer patients are heroic. My feeling is that heroism involves putting your life at risk to save that of another. The fireman who runs into a burning building to save a child is heroic. The passerby who stops and pulls a driver out of a burning car before the gas tank explodes is heroic. The citizen who stops a mugging or purse snatching is heroic. But cancer patients are not heroic in that sense. Some are courageous and brave in the face of adversity. And I am sure some are not. Two of the people I met early in this journey, I think of when I am feeling not so courageous.

The first is a man I met quite fortuitously when I was hospitalized last June from radiation sickness. When I was admitted he had not yet arrived. Another man with brain cancer was in the next bed. He was scheduled for surgery the next day. When I awoke that morning he was no longer my roommate but another had taken his place. Through the curtain separating the two bays, we spoke softly, but never face-to-face. He told me his name was Tom and when I heard the nurses call him Mr. Sawyer I couldn't help but laugh and asked him if that were truly his name. He laughed and said "yes" and laughed again when I told him that I had been an English teacher and had taught "his novel" several times. Together we laughed at the irony. Connection. We had connected over his name. And this faceless man became less invisible to me.

As the day progressed I realized Tom far worse than his cheerful voice belied; his condition far worse than my own. He would call for the nurses to bring him a bedpan, and when it did not arrive in a timely fashion, he softly uttered the words, "Too late". What followed was a flurry of activity. Nurses arrived. They struggled to lift Tom out of his bed, change his clothes, change his bed linens and clean him up This happened several times during the three days we were roommates. Not once did he get angry or frustrated with the nurses. Not once did he lose his temper. Not once did he apologize for soiling himself and having to be cleaned up. He remained with his dignity intact and never seemed to be demoralized.

When I had to pass by his bed to use the bathroom we said our first face-to-face hellos. Tom was a man of short stature, somewhat stocky, thick black hair and completely unable to move on his own. The nurses brought him his food and arranged it so that with his one good arm he could manage as best as possible to feed himself. His other arm was nearly totally blackened and looked near amputation. Tom had surrendered to his condition and had done so with dignity, pride and self-respect with no apologies for who he was or what was happening to him. I wished we had had more opportunity to talk, but he was heavily sedated and slept most of the day.

On the day I was discharged I stopped by his bed, shook his hand and told him that I had learned more from him about courage and bravery than I had from any other person or experience in my life. His simple thank you and smile were totally in character. I wished him good luck and left the room. I think of Tom Sawyer frequently and those thoughts give me strength to face my own adversities.

Thought For The Day

It is not what you gather, but what you scatter that tells you what kind of life you have lived.

Chapter 22

Today is a day of change. My port came out this AM and I am a 'free man'. It was the first time I have been out of this room in over a month — a mini-field trip downstairs to have the catheter removed. It felt good to wear regular clothes again. And the bald head doesn't look so bad when not dressed in a hospital gown all the time. I look somewhat normal — no wisecracks, please — until I have to wear a mask and gloves to venture out in public.

The second person who has had a profound effect on me was about three years old when I met him. During the four weeks of radiation treatments last summer I developed a severe case of vertigo and had to go to physical and occupational therapy. On several occasions, I shared the therapy room with this young boy and either his father or mother who had accompanied him. They were a young couple perhaps in their late 20's. Their son had been quite sick for most of his short life. His diagnosis I did not know, but it was some kind of cancer that affected his ability to walk and move about without assistance. He had that look, one that children of cancer often have, and one that is heart-wrenching. He was completely bald, skin the color of sun-bleached beach rocks, purple-blue veins readily visible though his paper thin skin. His eyes were sunken, and dark blue, almost eerie, yet always alert. And his smile never left his lips. He would struggle without his braces through the therapy exercises and wanted to do more when the session finished.

At first I thought his name was Duncan, which is kind of a cool name for a little kid. But write it off to radiation, vertigo, old age or the fact that his mom always had a cup of Dunkin' Donuts coffee in her hand. I came to learn that his real name was Griffin — an even cooler name for a little kid. So, in my mind he became Duncan-Griffin.

One particular morning Duncan-Griffin sat with his mom across from me in the waiting room. He had just come from chemo yet he was playful and energetic and just a bit impish. However, something was bothering him and his playfulness began to ebb. The smell of his mother's coffee in combination with the chemo was making him nauseous. Before he could make it to the men's room he got sick in the hallway leading to the therapy room. But like the soldier he had shown himself to be, he got up and let himself be cleaned off. He neither whined nor complained. He accepted what had happened and was ready to move on. Like his counterpart, Tom Sawyer, he lived with dignity and pride and acceptance of what was and never gave in or gave up. The strength of one so young, who has not known many healthy days in his life, was inspirational. The strength and courage of his parents was equally up-lifting. Without such caring parents, Duncan-Griffin might not have lived this long. They accepted the responsibility where many might have given up. They were truly noble.

Thought For The Day

---⊗⊗⊗---

The will of God will never take you where the grace of
God will not protect you.

CHAPTER 23

DAY T+24

After a less than a smooth transition into Hope Lodge last evening, I am finding myself enjoying my new found freedom. The downside of this freedom is that my body clock has not reset and it wakes me up for vitals and blood draws at midnight and again a 4 AM. The upside is that masked and gloved, I went downstairs and outside to get coffee this morning. The cool air felt so good. The coffee supremely good. Although I got the occasional strange look from some people, it was a pleasant maiden voyage. You know the old saying, "EFF-em if they can't take a joke!" Today I have to start fending for myself. All my needs are no longer being met. As I write this I have one load of laundry in the washing machine and another in the dryer. I made myself lunch. No more 'room service'. And life is good. So much is already behind me for which I am thankful, and so much more ahead, hopefully all good things.

I have a roommate. I did not want one, but Hope Lodge rules insist I have a "caretaker" 24-7. Tameka is my health care worker, a high-paid babysitter. She stays over during the week and returns on Mondays. She offers to do laundry and even cook. She is a kind-hearted person who truly loves her job. She is soft spoken and pretty much keeps to herself. I am not ungrateful, but I am also uncomfortable with sharing a relatively small living space with a stranger.

Thought For The Day

---∞∞∞---

Our greatest glory in not in never failing,
but in rising up every time we fail.

Ralph Waldo Emerson

CHAPTER 24

DAY T+ 25

I am now a quarter of the way through the first 100 days. In some ways it has gone quickly. Obviously, in others, not quickly enough.

Yesterday I made my dinner and ate in the kitchen-dining room. At Hope Lodge residents are required to eat in the communal kitchen and not in their own rooms. This fosters social interaction and diminishes isolation. It is a place to meet and converse with people and share our personal stories.

I met a man and his wife, Lew and Laurie, from Maryland. Lew was "stationed" on the 8th floor at Sloan, just down the hall from me. For a month we existed but yards away from each other and never knew. Lew was one day behind me in getting his transplant and was discharged from Sloan yesterday. Like me, he is totally bald, but he is thin. Lou lost his appetite and taste buds from the chemo and was just getting them back in the last couple of days. Laurie was making him what smelled like a delicious dinner. We ate at separate tables, and talked from across the room. It was comforting to have a comrade with similar experiences to compare notes. Days ago we did not know of each other's existence. Ironically, today our lives became enmeshed.

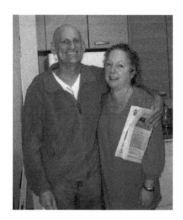

Lew and Laurie

This brings me to what I have learned in these last two days. For one, I've learned that God has a twisted sense of humor. Lew loses his appetite and taste buds and weight. Jim does not lose any of the above and gains weight, a lot of it. Aren't cancer patients supposed to lose weight and be thin? One for God. Zero for Jim.

I have lost all my hair. Bonus — saving on shampoo and conditioner. My beard, heavy enough to force me to shave in the morning and again if we were going out in the evening, has stopped growing. I haven't had to shave in three days. Bonus — saving on shaving cream. However, the hair in my ears and nose seem not to have gotten the same memo. Score: God - 2; Jim - 0.

Yesterday, when I went for my little three block walk, I thought I'd be cool. I put on my leather jacket, scarf, golf cap (damn, it's cold out there without any hair) and of course, the ever-present mask and blue gloves. To increase my coolness I flipped up the collar on my jacket, put a little strut in my walk and left Hope Lodge. As the final act of coolness I threw on my shades. I mean I was "all that and then some". However, and here's where God wins the no-contest match in a shutout, not more than four or five steps down the street my hot breath vs. the cold air was projected upward by the mask, fogging my glasses so much I couldn't see a blessed thing. God - 3; Jim - 0, final score. He/She knows how to bring you back to reality.

And maybe that is what this whole thing has been about — bringing me back to reality and what is really important.

Thought For The Day

The elevator to success is out of order.
You'll have to use the stairs one step at a time.

Joe Girardi

CHAPTER 25

The Good, the Bad and the Ugly redux

The Good:

Homemade chicken cutlet parmigiana dinners

An afternoon visit with my friend Flo. Non-stop conversation and laughter and tears and more laughter. Catching up is good. Learning new things about old friends — priceless.

A visit from Kristen and Mike

The much anticipated triumphal return of Nancy. Maybe even an unmasked kiss might be on the menu tonight.

My caretaker, Tameka. She is compassionate and most helpful. She looks after me like a doting mother. Her smile is disarming and immediately draws you into her kindness

Bone Marrow Aspiration on Thursday which will help determine how much my donor's stem cells have taken root. Technically, this could fit into the Ugly category as it is not a pleasant test. But, I'm being optimistic.

The Bad:

Blood levels of meds are low. Increased dose recommended

Constant 24/7 care mostly by strangers. No time to myself. I know. I was alone in the hospital wanting company I could not have. Now that I have constant care I want to be alone. Something about the grass being greener? Or is it God's sense of humor in action, again?

The Ugly:

Tameka's time with me ended and her replacement, "Hurricane Gloria", blew into town last Friday, all 4'11" of her packing verbal winds of 135-150 mph. A Category 4 itching to become a CAT 5. Yes, Gloria is a non-stop talker, unrelenting, savage! And when she wasn't talking she was watching Southern Baptist Bible shows on TV until the wee hours of the morning. I thought for sure there would be fire and brimstone raining down on me before she left. When I pretended to be a Buddhist, thinking that would end the proselytizing, the winds abated temporarily, only to return with the fury of the righteous having been scorned. Chapter and Verse were quoted about saving my damned soul.

On Saturday, I simply wanted to watch golf. I had missed Tiger's uneventful return in the match play last week. Although he was seven strokes behind Phil, I wanted to kick back in my less than comfortable non-recliner with a ginger ale, sans the Jack Daniels, some pretzels and watch the match. Gloria — who I prayed had blown out to sea, for she had been inordinately quiet all morning, perhaps due to all that late night soul saving — had moved out over the Hudson's warmer waters to gather strength, only to return as a CAT 5. From two o'clock to five o'clock she talked and talked and talked. Ironically, no one was listening, and yet she went on unabated. The visit from my daughter and sister provided shelter from the storm and I returned to the room about 9 PM took my nighttime meds and a double dose of Ambien and drifted into a calm, restful and quiet sleep.

In the morning, it seemed that Gloria had run out of steam and only the mere ghost of this former force remained. She asked for train fare home. In all fairness she had been ripped off by a cabbie who charged her $5 to take her the half block from Penn Station, and was short of cash. I gladly funded her departure and bid her fond farewell.

Thought For The Day

We cannot direct the wind, but we can adjust our sails.

CHAPTER 26

DAYS T+28, T+29 AND T+30

Today my morning at Sloan started at 8 AM and I got back to Hope Lodge at 2:30. Most of the day was again 'Hurry up and Wait'. Some things never change. The delays fed my paranoia. I was dreading the bone marrow aspiration. And God was working overtime. Surprise, surprise. I was scheduled for the aspiration and a bone marrow biopsy. The aspiration is not fun. However, the biopsy requires the extraction of a sizable chunk of marrow from my hip bone. This is tantamount to pulling a stubborn cork out of a wine bottle. If not enough marrow is extracted then in goes the needle again. The size of the needle is not to be spoken of in polite society. There is a loud popping sound that accompanies the extraction. The aspiration takes out a small amount of bone marrow fluid through a needle. Bone marrow biopsy uses a needle to take out bone with the marrow still inside it. The aspiration will confirm if the red blood cells are reproducing properly. The biopsy will confirm the presence of lymphoma in the bone marrow which would not be a good thing. The likelihood of this is slim as the past three aspirations have been negative and my numbers have been rising. The results should be available in three weeks and will tell how much of the bone marrow is mine and how much is my donor's. At this point I could be 100% my donor marrow, but more likely less because I declined the Neupogen shot. My DNA will change to his/hers as will my bone marrow. They will run the test for male or female bone marrow/DNA and that will determine how well the stem cells have done their job.

I must include this anecdote though at the time of the transplant I had no familiarity with Ancestry.com. My oldest granddaughter, Sophia, majored in digital forensics at Albany. I thought I would buy her and both my daughters Ancestry kits. When their results came in, my daughter, Kristen, called and asked if we were part Egyptian which had shown up in her results. Sophia had similar findings. Pretty sure that we are 100% Italian, we were all a bit confused. So I ordered a kit for myself. My results were startling. I was 0% Italian and a mixture of eastern European ethnicities. That a mistake had been made and my results were clearly incorrect, I called Ancestry. The representative asked if I were a match on my children's results or they on mine. In fact, I did not, recognize any of my matches. Nor was I a match for my children. The rep at Ancestry said she would investigate and get back to me. Two days later she called and asked if I had ever had a stem cell transplant. And therein lay the answer. My donor is apparently of eastern European decent. Originally my blood type was B+. My donor's was A+. For six months I would be chimeric — a combination of the two blood types — AB+ and then I will be totally A+. I also have her (yes, I found out my donor was female) DNA. Hence, nothing of the original me exists any longer. Having watched enough CSI and other forensic-based shows, I knew I could commit a crime and leave behind only female DNA. Hmmmm. Interesting plot line for an episode. The sad thing is that my golf buddies will not let me hit from the forward tees unless I shave my legs and wear a skirt and that ain't gonna happen!

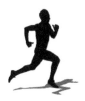

Thought For The Day

———∞∞∞———

I think men who have a pierced ear are better prepared
for marriage. They've experienced pain and bought
jewelry.

Rita Rudner

CHAPTER 27

DAY T+31 AND DAY T+32

Yesterday was the first day of Spring with its promise of warmer weather, and the greater promise of being sprung in a few weeks. And it was snowing! Something wrong with that picture.

It is amazing how we measure the passage of time. Some use the seasons — in two months it will be summer. Some simply use a watch or cell phone to mark the increments of time — "I have to pick up the kids in an hour". Others use special events or the anticipation of an event to measure time. — "We're leaving on vacation in 3 weeks. I can't wait". Or "I cannot believe my granddaughters are almost 6 and 10 years old. Where does the time go?"

But the transplant patient measures time in a different way. For example, the Day T+32 indicates I'm 32 days out of transplant or 68 days from being out of the danger zone. The other day at Sloan, I saw people who are where I was when I first met my oncologist and transplant team. And I realized how far I have come, which sometimes I lose sight of making progress in baby steps. Still I met others who were nearing their 100 day mark, still wearing masks and gloves, and mixing their chilled medications from their portable coolers, like I do, and realize how far I have yet to go.

Each day I go for walk and measure my progress of how far I can go without totally exhausting myself for the return trip. When I walk farther and for a longer time I know I am making progress and I set new goals for the next day.

When I go to the 12th floor's kitchen for a meal, I see empty spaces in the refrigerator — another way to measure the passing of time, I suppose. Another departure to the next leg of the trip? A death? I see new bins filled with new food indicating a new arrival. And the cycle continues.

Lisa is the young woman who lives across the hall from me. She may be the 'owner' of the new food bin. She is perhaps 40 but seems much younger, almost child-like. She is of frail build, short dark hair, pale complexion and dark eyes that never make real eye contact. She speaks rarely and only in muted, mumbled tones, barely audible. Like the Chief in Ken Kesey's <u>One Flew Over the Cuckoo's Nest</u>, Lisa regularly sweeps the kitchen eating area in silence. It seems to give her purpose. She is frightened and alone. She has no caretaker and I have never seen her with any visitors. She is quite sick from all the radiation she is getting and Hope Lodge may ask her to leave if she cannot find someone to stay with her. She is another face of cancer and one by which I have come to measure my progress during the time I have spent here.

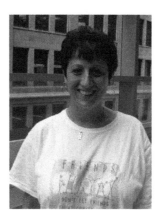

Lisa

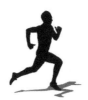

Thought For The Day

Not everything that counts can be counted, and not everything that can be counted counts.

Albert Einstein

CHAPTER 28

DAY T+33

I am one-third the way home.

Many nice things happened yesterday. I had the good fortune to spend part of the day with friends from the theater, Kathy and George. It was good to see them after such a long absence. They brought news of the outside world and catching up was just the best medicine. I apologize to several of you for not remembering important things happening in your lives because, honestly, I have been so caught up in my own stuff, that I forgot there is another whole world going on outside. Perhaps this is one of those things that I needed to learn —

Note to self: be more aware of others and not so self-absorbed.

Another nice thing happened today. Hurricane Gloria called. Despite my somewhat harsh treatment of her in earlier postings, she called to tell me that she had prayed for me last Sunday at church and all week long and will do so again tomorrow. My momma didn't raise no fool. If someone wants to pray for me, I will graciously accept those prayers, even if they are from Gloria. Hell, it can't hurt. Not going to look a gift prayer in the mouth.

Today is a day of great anticipation. First, I am going to see my granddaughter, Sophia, for the first time in nearly two months. It is going to be so hard not to hug her with great big Poppa hugs. Kristen and Mike are coming to spend the afternoon and then Nancy arrives later and will stay through Tuesday. Now if that ain't hittin' the jackpot, I don't know what is.

Thought For The Day

---∞∞∞---

Count your age by your friends.
Count your life by your smiles.

Day T+34 T+35 and T+36

I haven't been on the computer much these last few days. Real people take precedence. My visit with Kristen and Mike and the lovely and talented Ms. Sophia was joyful. In the last two months since I've seen her, she has grown physically, intellectually and emotionally. I have missed watching her grow and being a part of it. She whipped Poppa's butt in Wii Bowling and I declined her challenge to play Wii golf or tennis. Enough humiliation for one day. When did she get so good? When did she become so beautiful? When did she grow so tall? "Sunrise, Sunset". I vowed not to let this disease rob me of any more of these precious times.

Nan arrived on Sunday evening and left yesterday and that is always a pleasure — not her leaving but rather her staying for more than a few hours. We still laugh a lot and share so many wonderful moments together after all these years. The laughter makes me forget even for the briefest moment why I am here.

Clarification: Many have asked where Meals on Wheels of Bluepoint is located. My veiled attempt at humor has fallen flat on its face and in the process, my sister, Susan, who lives in Bluepoint and who makes and delivers these great home cooked meals to me, is not getting the credit she deserves. In fact she is due this evening with a pork chop dinner that she says will blow my mind. No doubt that it will. Her track record is impeccable.

Results from my blood work are good and preliminary results from the bone marrow aspiration showed that the stem cells are doing their job. Three weeks more and I will find out if there is any lymphoma recurrence. Of course, these, the most significant results, are the ones I have to wait for the longest. Ain't that always the case?

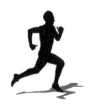

Thought For The Day

All human wisdom is summed up in two words —
wait and hope.

Alexandre Dumas

CHAPTER 29

DAY T+37

The kitchen the 12th floor of Hope Lodge (each residence floor has its own) is the gathering spot at mealtimes for the floor's locals who cook their meals. We are not allowed to eat in our rooms as I've mentioned, for hygienic as well as social interaction reasons. Since I cannot eat at restaurants yet, this is where I find myself three times a day.

It is in this kitchen that I have met some unbelievable people whose stories are moving and uplifting and devastating all at the same time. I have spoken of Lisa already. She is still here but her "disappearance" for several days has had most of us concerned. We have become an extended family of sorts. We look out for each other. Comrades in arms. After one of her clinic visits, Lisa had to be hospitalized for a heart arrhythmia. However, when she returned to the 12th she seemed better both physically and mentally. She still has no caregiver. Her brother simply drops her off on Sunday after a weekend in New Jersey. Over the last several days Lisa has become more involved in conversations and the goings-on in the kitchen. But yesterday, as my sister and I were leaving to go on our walk, Lisa emerged from her room in tears. One of her dear friends had lost her battle with cancer. Lisa was devastated, inconsolable. She just cannot seem to catch a break. News of this kind smacks us all in the face with our mortality. None of us is immune to it. And it creates anxiety in all of us.

Another denizen of the communal dining area is the Kitchen Dominatrix. I've already used Nazi as in the Urine Nazi, so I had to find another descriptor. I don't know this woman's name, or her husband's — he is the patient. KD enters the kitchen in a whirlwind of commotion and seeks out any violations or infractions of Hope Lodge's rules. She cleans every area before and after using it and audibly "tsk-tsks" about how negligent people are. She is a self-admitted clean freak who, so I have heard, has been known to chastise others for leaving crumbs on the table or not washing utensils in a timely fashion. I had the occasion to share a lunch table with KD and her husband, Mr. KD, a Casper Milquetoast type who has undergone several years of treatment and multiple surgeries. KD finished all his sentences for him and even answered questions I had posed directly to him. She seemed to have little faith in the choices the doctors at Sloan had offered for his treatment and felt that his prognosis was poor. She expressed these sentiments and doubts in front of him which I found most disconcerting. However, in my quest to become less judgmental of people, I came to understand that she was frightened. She had no control over what was happening to her husband or to her or to their lives. The only thing she could control was the conversation and the cleanliness of the kitchen. When she spoke somewhat lovingly of the pre-cancer times in their lives and how those days might never be recaptured, a great sense of loss crept into her eyes. When I came to understand this, it made me sad. It reinforced the idea that this disease tries to seize control of everything from us and we must fight not to relinquish it. It is not an easy fight for some.

I did, however, make sure I cleaned up my spot after lunch.

I will speak more of the kitchen characters later but I want to end this chapter on one of the highlights of my stay in NYC.

Yesterday, as Susan and I left for our walk up 7th Ave toward Penn Station, a man in a grey three-piece pinstriped business suit, laptop and briefcase in hand, caught up to us and walked beside us for a bit. He pointed at my mask and gloves and said, "I used to dress like you two years ago. Then I had a stem cell transplant for leukemia. It works. Good luck to you." Whoa! How incredible was that? A perfect stranger. In NYC. There are good people in this world. As quickly as he spoke to us, he disappeared into the crowd of commuters. And as hard as I tried to visually follow him I could not. He seemed to disappear into thin air. Many have told me this was an 'angel sighting'. I like that and I think I will run with that explanation.

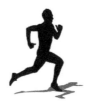

Thought For The Day

---⎯∞∞⎯---

The roots of all goodness lie in the soil of appreciation
for goodness.

Dalai Lama

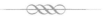

CHAPTER 30

DAY T+ 38

I met Lee and Terry probably at the end of January or the beginning of February while at Sloan for one of my many pre-transplant tests. They sat opposite me in the waiting room and as is wont to happen, we struck up a conversation. The common bond of cancer patients is a mighty one. All the fears and concerns that are sometimes not expressed to our doctors are shared, ironically, with perfect strangers. I found out that Lee was going for pre-op tests for a hip transplant and this how his cancer was discovered. It struck me as odd because my mother's cancer was detected in much the same way. The testing for a rather commonplace surgery led to the discovery of something far more serious. Fortunately, in Lee's case, this discovery would save his life. He is about two weeks behind me in his transplant date. We nearly share the same "re-birth-day".

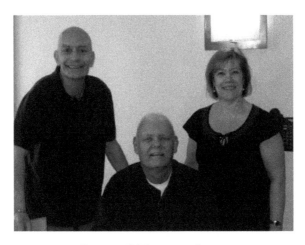

Lee and Terry and me

As things would have it, they are also a part of the 12th floor clan with whom I share meals, conversation, questions and concerns. They have become part of my extended family. Two nicer people you could not ask to have as "accidental friends". Lee has a feistiness and a fight in him that won't let him quit. He inspires me. Terry is kind and gentle. It is obvious why their marriage has lasted 38 years. They are the yin to the other's yang. A perfect compliment to one another. They adore one another. Their goodness and his grit spill over onto the rest of us. I am most thankful we have met.

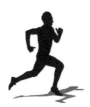

Thought For The Day

———∞∞∞———

Nothing is accidental in the universe — this is one of
my Laws of Physics — except the entire universe itself,
which is Pure Accident, pure divinity

Joyce Carol Oates

CHAPTER 31

Day T+39

Jackie and her husband have been here for over a year while he is being treated. I have not met him because he stays in his room and she brings him his meals, contrary to Hope Lodge rules, yet with good reason. He has esophageal cancer, has had numerous radiation treatments and can hardly swallow and keep food down due to the massive scarring. They started his treatments well over a year ago, and were staying at the Helmsley Hotel in NYC at a cost of $10,000 a month. When their funds ran out they had to declare bankruptcy and they moved to the YMCA. Conditions at the Y were not conducive to his healing and so they found their way here. Cancer does not care about your finances. It just plows ahead with little regard for how, or if, you can afford treatment.

Jackie is the Kitchen Matron, all 5' 2" of her. She knows the workings of Hope Lodge inside and out and has stayed on just about every floor here. Unlike KD (the dominatrix) Jackie embodies the spirit of the name of this place — HOPE. Her strength is incredible. When all seems to be lost she, the caretaker, has not lost hope. She tells us stories of days gone by as if we were her children or grandchildren. She is passing down a history of sorts. And while her husband's disease is unlike any of ours, we sit and pay her due respect for all that she has endured and overcome.

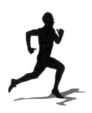

Thought For The Day

---∞∞∞---

Once you choose hope, anything's possible.

Christopher Reeve

CHAPTER 32

Stuart and Barbara are prime examples of how one must play the hand one has been dealt. Barbara has had polio from age 9. She wears a leg brace which goes from her hip to her ankle. Although she is mobile, she is at times unsteady necessitating a wheelchair if she must go long distances. She is bright, amiable and sociable and a bit younger than I am. At first I thought she was the patient. But ironically, Barbara's husband, Stuart is the patient and she his caretaker. While Stuart can be a little rough around the edges, he has a sharp sense of humor. Stuart served in Viet Nam in the late 60's and early 70's and was discharged in 1973. During one dinnertime conversation he asked me, "What are you in for?" I told him and returned the question. Thirty years after his discharge, in 2003 he was diagnosed with leukemia. My doctors do not know what causes non-Hodgkins lymphoma, but Stuart knew what had caused his leukemia — exposure to Agent Orange while in Nam. It lay dormant for three decades and then surfaced when least expected. The aces and eights hand.

The other day Stuart had an appointment at Sloan and he and Barbara decided to take the bus instead of a cab. So there they were, Barbara and Stuart — she with polio, he with leukemia; Barbara in her wheelchair and Stuart pushing her from behind. When the bus handicap ramp was lowered to accommodate her, Stuart lost his balance, grabbed hold of the handle of Barbara's wheelchair sending them both toppling to the pavement. So what did they do? They got up brushed themselves off, got on the bus and went about their business. And that is what we do. Sometimes we fall but we get up. There really is no other choice. The trick, as someone once said, is to get up one more time than you fall.

Causes. For someone like me who has this need to know "why", not knowing the cause of my cancer has proven very difficult. Some conjecture that it was stress. I can go with that. With my type A personality I accept that explanation. Perhaps when my donor's DNA takes over and my blood type changes from B+ to A+ maybe my personality will go from Type A to Type B. Some say that lymphoma is brought on by the pesticides and fertilizers seeping in the ground water. Still others contend the source of the cancer can be found in the preservatives in our food. None of that definitively answers the question "why?" If I were told I had lung cancer then I could see the correlation — you chose to smoke for so many years you get lung cancer. Read the warning on the side of the pack of cigarettes, dummy! But with NHL there is no cause and effect link between the two. As many people who never smoked get NHL, as those who did smoke. The question bores deeply. What am I being punished for? What have I done that was so horrible to deserve this? I have heard that this is a common question of even those who know the cause of their cancer. But for those who do not, particularly me, it is a constant nagging, though it is growing less and less as time passes. Maybe it is just that I have had to learn to play the cards I have been dealt, to be flexible to surrender to what I cannot change, and to fight with dignity what I can. To be more like Barbara and Stuart.

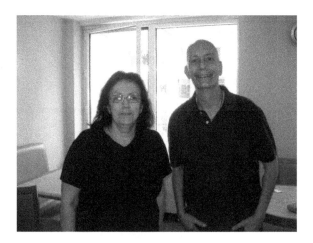

Barbara and me

None of this is to say that I am feeling sorry for myself at all. I was more focussed on the idea of us playing the hand we are dealt. The fact that I have cancer is not going to change by knowing what caused it. It would only help me understand. Show me how you do the magic trick and it demystifies the illusion. And I grow from that understanding.

Thought For The Day

―――――――∞∞∞―――――――

We learn more by looking for the answer to a question and
not finding it than we do from learning the answer itself.

Lloyd Alexander

Day T+41

On Thursday I should get the results of the bone marrow biopsy and maybe a hint of when I might be paroled. I miss home so much. I am registered here until April 15th but my stay might have to be extended. In reality, my 100 days are not up until May 28th. Many of my kitchen cohorts are here for the full 100 days. Their circumstances and distances from home vary from mine so I am trying not to use them as my yardstick.

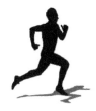

Thought For The Day

---ᗞᗞᗞ---

Judge a man by his questions rather than by his answers.

Voltaire

CHAPTER 33

DAYS T+42 T+43 AND T+44

I post this news with guarded optimism after my appointment with Dr. Perales. Though he has yet to confer with the team, what I heard or wanted to hear was most encouraging. First, my counts are good. A few are still a bit low but not of major concern. I look healthy and I am exercising and walking a mile+ a day when the weather is good. Bone marrow is clear of the lymphoma and I am 96% chimeric. All indications are that the transplant was successful. I still have to be cautious for the next eight months, but I got the green light to go to my daughter's wedding in July without mask or gloves. Back in February, I grabbed Dr. Perales by the lapels of his lab coat, startling him. I told him he had to keep me alive until at least July 6 so I could walk my daughter down the aisle. Of course he couldn't promise anything, but assured me that he would try. I still have to be careful about sun exposure as it can kick off graft vs host disease and my body might begin to reject the transplant. And it is a beach wedding. So sunscreen, hat and then early morning/late afternoon tee times only. But all those are small asks. The best news is that it is looking good for my coming home on April 15th. That will put me at Day T+57. I have been away far too long.

With that good news I went on what was to be my last grocery shopping at Gristede's and walked the half mile home with two bagsful. While in the cereal aisle I excused myself past a shopper in one of those motorized chairs. As I passed, she stopped me and asked, "Why are you wearing that mask?" Several smart-ass answers came to mind but I told her the simple truth — "I am a stem cell transplant cancer patient and immuno-suppressed." She was afflicted with MS. There is a camaraderie that binds those who are fighting some kind of battle. We spoke for several minutes. Connection is such a powerful force. It makes one feel less invisible. It strengthens one's resolve and inspires one to keep fighting.

When I returned to Hope Lodge several of my kitchen mates awaited my good news. Their joy was only eclipsed by my own. It is wonderful when those who know what you have endured through first-hand experience, celebrate with you!

Thought For The Day

Put yourself in a state of mind where you say to yourself, "Here is an opportunity for me to celebrate like never before, my own power my own ability to get myself to do what is necessary."

Anthony Robbins

CHAPTER 34

DAYS T+45, T+46, T+47, T+48, T+49 AND T+50

Today I am halfway through my 100 days. Seven more weeks and the risk of developing graft vs host diminishes significantly.

Yesterday was a long day. I had a four-hour infusion of meds for GVHD, and then I was tented again for termites as per my exterminating contract!

Last week I said I was guardedly optimistic about my parole date. Well, it turns out that "guarded" was the operative word. Despite everything the doctor told me last week and how high my spirits were when I left the hospital, yesterday's news was at best discouraging. While my counts are up and I am feeling well enough to go home and start living some semblance of a normal life, the doctor who calls the shots sent his nurse (I think he might have been afraid of my reaction to deliver the news himself) to tell me that I cannot go home until at least day T+75 and even that is not is stone. "He normally does not release patients until day T+90," she added. Since the nurse was the harbinger of bad news, and it is not polite to shoot the messenger, I did not have the chance to ask the doctor, "Why?" There's that nagging question again. Why, if all my counts are up, and I am feeling healthy, looking healthy and the bone marrow biopsy results were good, why am I not able to go home? I am not one who deals easily with the response, "Because I said so." If you could ask my parents they would bear that out. But it seems that with no other answer,

"Because I said so" seems to be the only explanation I'm going to get until I see him on Tuesday. And then he will have some 'splainin' to do, Lucy!

When I returned to the 12th floor my kitchen comrades were eager to hear my good news and they were as disappointed for me now as they are overjoyed for me last week. Each reflected on his/her own fate and the possible postponement of parole. The room echoed the many unanswered questions and the uncertainties we were all feeling. Once again, this accidental family was bonding and rallying around someone going through a rough time. This is what this disease does. In the end we were all laughing, well, smiling at least, even if it were only at ourselves and our frailties. As I left the kitchen Laurie said to me, "For as long as you have to stay, we will make you laugh."

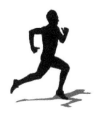

Thought For The Day

───⟨∞∞∞⟩───

Disappointment to a noble soul is what cold water is to
burning metal; it strengthens, tempers intensifies, but
never destroys it."

Eliza Tabor

CHAPTER 35

DAY T+56

Well, all good things must come to an end and my stay here at Hope Lodge is no exception. This morning Dr. Perales gave me the OK to go home at the end of the week. While I am not happy about the delay, I understand the "why" (there's that ugly word again) and I am ok with the postponement. Many of my medications were changed to tablet form. This is far more convenient than the liquid, draw-up-in-a-syringe-and-keep-refrigerated-when-not-in-use kind. My body will have to adjust to these. Other meds have been discontinued. Rather than risk a reaction to the new dosages, it would be better to be close by over the next week and a half in case something should happen or adjustments need to be made. All said and done, I should be back at the ranch by day T+67 — two thirds the way through the risk period.

As odd as this may sound, I am going to miss some things about this place. For one, my "accidental family" will be sorely missed, in particular, Terry and Lee. They have become dear friends. Cancer makes for strange bedfellows. Lee is an ultraconservative Republican and Terry is as well, I'm sure. Under normal circumstances, we might not have much in common and would not have spoken more than pleasantries had we attended the same get-together, which in and of itself would be highly unlikely. But we have a common bond now. I am learning to be less judgmental and more accepting. Lee has shown a side of himself to me that he might not risk showing his other friends. Both he and Terry are supportive and sympathetic and kind. We can joke with each other. Lee teases about my female DNA and I find myself going right along with it. He has blue eyes which twinkle when he is about to zing me, giving me just enough time to duck. Man, I'd love to get him in a poker game. At first, Terry did most of the talking for them both. It took Lee a little more time to feel comfortable opening up. And but for fate, we might have never met.

What I shall not miss is the topics of conversation in the kitchen. There are so many new people on the floor who are where we all were a month ago. The talk revolves around cancer and the dreadful stories about treatments and side effects. And though once I participated in these discussions, I now find them deeply saddening and need to distance myself from them. I listen with a sympathetic, supportive ear, knowing that there but for the grace of God go I, but I need to surround myself with more positive energy.

Thought For The Day

———⚇———

We should come home from adventures, and perils, and discoveries every day with new experience and character.

Henry David Thoreau

DAY T+58

Another reason I need to go home … Yesterday Lisa seemed to be doing quite well. She was laughing and enjoying the conversation. For the first time in many weeks she seemed to be emerging from her shell. Her treatment regimen has been difficult at best. She goes for chemo for six hours every Monday and then radiation the rest of the week. She still has no caregiver; no family visits her. The chemo and radiation have caused severe side effects that have wreaked havoc with her digestive system. Here at Hope Lodge, because of the economy and cutbacks in corporate donations, we are limited to two rolls of toilet paper per week and Lisa is constantly running out. We have all chipped in giving her our extra or buying some for her. Talk about stripping away one's dignity! But yesterday, she was laughing and even gave us a fashion show with her new wig. Lisa's hair is short and dark brown but her wig is shoulder length and auburn, something she treated herself to facing the inevitability of losing all her hair. One of the things cancer patients must learn is how to self-soothe. This is not always easy. Some feel they don't deserve to be soothed; others are too tired or too sick to be bothered; and still others don't know how. But it must be done. And so we laughed along with Lisa and suggested new screen names for her like "Red Hot Mama".

Today, however, Lisa came into the kitchen a completely different person. She was pale and drawn. No wig. No smile. No conversation. It was as if someone had slipped in during the night and stolen her spirit. She was sick and visibly shaking. Her sunken eyes, ringed with dark circles, seemed as if they were about to roll up into her head. Her treatments and new meds were getting the best of her. It was Lee who noticed her condition and at our insistence, Lisa gave in to being taken to the hospital. She looked so alone, so frightened and so sick. Terry volunteered to go with her by taxi not only to make sure she would be all right, but also not to raise suspicions that she had no caretaker and would have to leave Hope Lodge. They were just two girls going on a shopping spree. Returning alone, Terry told us that Lisa would be kept overnight for observation and treatment.

I cannot imagine doing this by myself, alone, sick and scared. It saddens me deeply to see another human being suffering so.

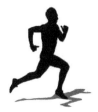

Thought For The Day

Instead of comparing our lot with that of those who are more fortunate than we are, we should compare it with the great majority of our fellow men. It then appears that we are among the privileged

Helen Keller

CHAPTER 36

DAY T+61

Friday I had two doctor appointments; the morning for blood draws — CBC and med levels. For the afternoon appointment I arrived 15 minutes early and waited 2 hours in the appropriately named "waiting room" and then another 15 minutes in the examining room before seeing the doctor. I know we have all been there and waiting is not unusual for an oncology appointment. But what really gets my shorts in a knot is when the doctor comes in, does the virtual handshake seeing my mask and gloves, which I have been wearing for seven and a half hours, pulls up my files and for ten minutes reads me the notes Dr. Perales entered. He examines me for five minutes and says, "Everything is ok. Make a follow up appointment in six months. I'll make a copy of your new meds." I'm sure while he was doing this he was also billing the insurance company for hundreds of dollars for this appointment. Hmmm.... health care reform? No wonder medical costs have risen.

Back at Hope Lodge I had lunch with my sister and later that evening I had the great fortune of IM'ing my 9 year old granddaughter. If anything could make the waste of the afternoon hours disappear, it is time spent with her — even in cyberspace. She is such a delight and, regardless of my mood, she makes me smile. She is the best medicine by far. Science should bottle her enthusiasm, her humor and her intelligence and give all patients an IV drip of Sophia.

Yesterday I took full advantage of the beautiful weather, walked down to Chelsea Piers, rented a driver, a 5 iron, a pitching wedge, and a bucket of balls and hit away for an hour. For my golf buddies, best beware. You will have to carry a calculator to figure out how many strokes you are going to have to give me per hole. But, hell, I was outdoors and swinging a golf club. What could be better?

Mask Mishaps and Gloved Gaffs

I know I have mentioned people's reactions to my walking the streets of NYC donning a mask and gloves. People stare at the mask and when I make eye contact with them, they avert my glance, looking down only to find themselves staring at the gloves. Then they look back up and find I'm still staring at them. Makes them uncomfortable, but it is how I amuse myself.

The other day I was in K-Mart and a woman looked at me and said, "Oh my. That is scary. Should I be wearing one of those too?" and then she quickly disappeared behind the racks of Easter bunnies. Another such encounter was with a cashier in Duane Reade (I hang out in really swanky stores, if you haven't noticed). She kept staring at me as she rang up my purchases. When I could no longer take her worrisome stare, I finally said to her, "Child, I'm not going to rob you or ask you to hand over all the cash in your register. I'm just here to buy toothpaste and deodorant." Hands on hips she rolled her eyes, in a fashion not unlike my children used to do being caught doing something inappropriate.

But the best two encounters happened within 24 hours of each other. I was in Borders (yes, I was social climbing) at about 9:15 PM. The cashier, a young girl of no more than 22-23 years, wearing far too much make-up and snapping gum, stared at my mask and gloves. Unable to contain herself she asked, "Are you a doctor?" My first reaction, (I'm learning to control the impulse to be snarky and answer more seriously) was, "No, but I play one on TV." However, I refrained and simply explained that I had cancer, was immuno-suppressed and wore my "costume" to protect me from infection. All of this fell on deaf and disappointed ears. She pouted. Her heavily lipsticked lower lip quivered somewhat, and said, "I wanted to ask you about my gallstones and whether you think I should have surgery?" Undeterred, she persisted in her quest for medical advice despite my attempts to shrug her off. The only way to get out of this uncomfortable situation and the store itself was to give her something to chew on so I suggested she get a second opinion. Oh boy! And she will be paying my social security for years to come. Ah, life on the outside.

The last encounter occurred when I was walking home from Chelsea Piers. As I walked up 8th Ave. though masked and gloved, I was not wearing a hat, letting the cool April air caress my bald head. On each street corner people were giving handouts to passersby usually advertising one service or another or a lap dance at some strip club. But not this time. When I looked down at the handbill I could not help but laugh and the man who had just handed it to me, couldn't figure out why. It was for a haircut and a shave. Yes, they walk among us.

Thought For The Day

---⬡⬡⬡---

Laughter is an orgasm triggered by the intercourse of
sense and nonsense.

CHAPTER 37

DAY T+ 64 OR DAY H-4 HOME IN 4 DAYS!

After two and a half months, it looks like I am finally going to go home on Saturday. I must pass a few more blood tests and the most concerning is the fluctuating neutrophil levels which indicate how capable my white blood cells are in fighting infection. The fluctuation might be due to the new meds and med levels and my body not having completely adjusted to them. I remain optimistic. Only when I am in the car headed east on the Long Island Expressway will I believe it is actually happening.

Quick update on a few people who have haunted these pages previously.

Lisa: I don't know how much more this woman can take. She has got major heart problems now. After her hospitalization last week, when her heart rate was sky high, she now needs a pacemaker. On top of her full hysterectomy last fall, her mother's death from cancer in October and now her own chemo and radiation, she has run out of sick time to get her through the end of her radiation treatments. Not realizing her employer miscalculated her sick time, she did not apply for disability. She might lose her job, have no viable source of income and no one to take care of her. I suggested she to speak with her social worker or a patient advocate. Cancer has robbed her, and many like her, of her job, her well-being and her dignity. Cancer's effect is not just physical.

Lee: Lee's counts have dropped significantly and the doctor has him on four days of anti-graft-vs-host IVs. Each treatment is four hours long. Cancer patients usually get only one a month. The doctors feel it might be that the new bone marrow may not like his new meds, or a virus has infected his blood, or that his body is rejecting the stem cells. I am so concerned. To be this far out of transplant and have it possibly fail, is of grave consequence. This could easily happen to me as well. It is far too much to wrap my brain around now. We are both scared.

Stuart: His leukemia has had him in and out of the hospital with pneumonia and a severe reaction to the "joy juice" as he calls his chemo. This morning he was rushed by ambulance to Sloan. No word on his condition so far. But Lisa, who has enough problems of her own, was concerned because she had his jacket he let her hold when he left. She was worried he might need it and she would have no way to get it to him. Amazing. All of us maintain a high level of hope that laces its way though our fears, anxieties and worries. We jump in to support one another whenever we can. We, the accidental friends of Floor 12.

Thought For The Day

I have learned two lessons in my life: first, there are no
sufficient literary psychological or historical answers to
human tragedy, only moral ones. Second, just as despair
can come to one another only from other human
beings, hope, too, can be given to one only by other
human beings.

Elie Wiesel

CHAPTER 38

DAY T+66 DAY H-1

Two-thirds the way through the danger period. Well, almost.

"All my bags are packed. I'm ready to go…" and although I won't be leaving on a jet plane a certain beautiful, Swedish blonde is scheduled to pick me up tomorrow at 11 AM in my blue Volvo convertible for the trip HOME! Blood work is fine; meds do not need to be tweaked; no Neupogen shot needed. The human body is an amazing machine that I have come to appreciate so much in the course of the last two and a half months. It is incredible what it is designed to do and how it is able to accomplish those tasks. Sprinkle with some meds and an overdose of hope and positivity and it will soar. I am ready to soar and I am ready to go HOME. Did I mention that already?

My thoughts today are running wild and in a million different directions. Forgive the randomness of this post.

Lisa is much better today. She looks good, said she feels good and is going home this weekend to return next week for her final 3 radiation treatments. All got squared away with her job. This morning she came to my room with a gift bag and a card in her hand. I was overwhelmed. The gift — a coffee mug with words of inspiration inscribed; the card a message, that I had the foresight to read privately because, as you can well-imagine, reduced me to a blathering idiot, simply said, "I believe".

While at Sloan getting the last of my blood draws, a woman opposite me in the lab was quite squeamish and the hematologist was having a difficult time getting her to sit still enough for him to start. She kept insisting she hated needles. The hematologist, with a gentle sense of humor, pointed out the irony of her protests, drawing attention to the numerous tattoos she had on her arm. You just gotta laugh.

Another man waiting for his monthly follow-up visit approached me and asked when I had had my transplant — the mask and gloves a dead giveaway. He was coming up on his year anniversary and looked great. I learned from our conversation that he was 39 years old and had four children under the age of 8. I could not imagine when, as he told me that he almost died this year due to an infection, what impact his death would have had on his young family. He had just returned home from a trip to Disney with his children and as he so pointedly said, "I cannot waste a minute of this chance I have been given."

I am leaving tomorrow with mixed feelings. I am thrilled to be going home. Yet there is some fear. I hope this time's the charm. I also leave with some guilt feelings about those I am leaving behind. I am the first of our group to be pardoned. I know the time for the others will come, and I pray they come sooner than later. My friend Terri White asked me, "Is there psychological/emotional support therapy for patients when they reenter the real world. It is much like a PTSD or survivor guilt scenario transitioning from one life to another and leaving others behind?" Her point is well-taken. I am entering a whole new phase of recovery, one that I hope I can ease into without much difficulty.

For those who do not know, the Leukemia Lymphoma Society has a wonderful program that helps both patients, caregivers and their families adjust. They pair people with those who have the same kind of cancer. As a first connect person with the Society, I have met and spoken with more than a dozen such patients. It gives patients about to start or who are already in treatment the chance to speak with someone who has already been there. As helpful as I would like to think I was, I received as much from speaking with others similarly affected as I hope they did from talking with me. I am sure there are other organizations other than the Leukemia Lymphoma Society which deal with specific kinds of cancers which can be most helpful.

Thought For The Day

sent to me by my cousin,
Bobbie and her daughter, Laura

May today there be peace within.
May you trust that you are exactly where you are meant
to be.
May you not forget the infinite possibilities that are
born of faith in yourself an others.
May you use the gifts you have received, and pass on the
love that has been given to you.
May you be content with yourself just the way you are.
Let this knowledge settle in your bones an allow your
soul the freedom to sing, dance, praise and love.
It is there for each and every one of us.

CHAPTER 39

DAY T+71 DAY H+0

Home Sweet Home!

Oh, Auntie Em, Auntie Em. There's no place like home. There's no place like home.

So, this beautiful Swedish lady arrived on Saturday, top down (on the car— get your mind out of the gutter) and whisked me away from Hope Lodge in 85+ degree temperatures. The drive home was liberating. The forsythia along the LIE was in full bloom. There was green grass, not cement, wherever I looked. And with the top down the wind tousled my hair. OK, I got a little carried away for a moment. I can dream, can't I? A better homecoming I could not have asked for. My daughter and Mike had strung a mylar "Welcome Home" banner across my front windows to herald the "prodigal son's return".

My departure from Hope Lodge was not without difficulty. Saying goodbye to the dear friends I had made over the last six weeks was fraught with mixed emotions. We all had fought different battles in the same war. We did so with dignity and strength and support from each other. We laughed and shed tears and shared private moments. Sometimes it was depressing and sapped my energy. But mostly I laughed. Even at the gallows humor. If I had to be holed up with a rag-tag group, I would choose to be with these people again.

Now that I am home, it will take time to re-acclimate to this new found freedom. The concern over which cabinet my drinking glasses and silverware were brought both frustration and a smile. Now I must deal with traffic, paying bills, picking up my mail, going food shopping — all the pedestrian things of day to day living — the operative word being 'living'. Unpacking the car I was surprised, not sure why, to see my winter jacket, sweaters, gloves, scarves. I had not paid much attention when packing to come home. Now they seemed odd and out of place in the summer-like weather. They marked the passage of time. Had it really been two and a half months? Had I really been gone that long? The winter clothes said, "Yes".

Yesterday I had my first blood draws at Sloan since coming home. A two an a half hour trip plus a 40 minute wait to get into the hospital's parking garage made me 20 minutes too late for the draws and I was told to go home and return in the morning. Despite the nearly five hours' driving time yesterday and much road rage, largely in the form of very foul language, it is done for another week.

A reunion with neighbors and friends, whose sincere happiness at my return was more than just therapeutic. It was heartwarming. So, yes, it is good to be home, Auntie Em.

Thought For The Day

I'm still standing, but I'm not standing still.

me

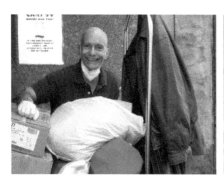 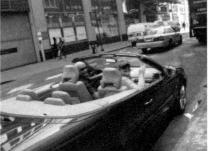

CHAPTER 40_

Three Quarters through the Danger Zone — with all due apologies to Kenny Loggins

When I walk through a public place, masked and gloved, people see me and purposely steer clear of my path, assuming I am contagious or infectious. One person found the courage to question whether I was overdoing the precaution thing. When I told her it was more to protect me from her than her from me, there was a deafening silence and in its awkwardness, I managed to escape. One young mother, child in tow, saw me round the corner into her aisle of the supermarket, did a quick about face and beat a hasty retreat as far from this scary and possibly dangerous man. I am learning about prejudice through people's ignorance.

Despite my counts rising, the anxiety over my upcoming PET and CT scans is growing. For those of you who have battled or are battling cancer or who have been caretakers, you know that this will be part of our lives forever. I do not have a good track record with first-follow-up scans, having relapsed three times. I anxiously await the May 21 and May 22 tests. I am not sure how to handle this with anything but guarded optimism. I seem to operate in that mode often.

There is more to say but not much of it is happy. Since my departure from Hope Lodge I have kept in touch with my accidental family. My weekly appointments at Sloan coincide with Lee's and it is always good to see him and Terry. Privately, Terry told me Lee is not doing well. His counts are dropping, despite a change in his meds and four days of graft vs host infusions. Dropping counts sometimes indicate rejection. Lee is only two weeks behind me in transplant time so today he is T+67. I guess for at least a year we will live on the edge of anxiety.

The worst news from Hope Lodge is that Marsha passed away last night. She had to be the most optimistic person on the 12th floor. When I first met her, I thought she was the caregiver and her husband, Jim, the patient. She was quick with a smile and her eyes twinkled as she nightly made plans for the next day's trip. Marsha and Jim are from Greensboro, SC and being out-of-staters, she did not want to waste the opportunity of being in the Big Apple. I wonder if she 'knew' as some say the dying do. They did all the touristy things and each night would return in time for her to cook dinner, plan their excursions for the next day and download recipes for the next night's meal. In time, Marsha's pain confined her to a wheelchair, her face showed the toll it was taking on her body, but her spirit never faltered.

Eventually she was hospitalized at St. Vincent's, ironically the hospital where I was born. Jim moved out of Hope Lodge to spend their last few nights together. I learned that the doctors in Greensboro had given up on her and had told her there was nothing more they could do. But Marsha never gave up hope. She fought her pancreatic cancer. She fought through the pain, and I am sure she fought until the moment she could fight no more. The screen in front of me is blurry now so I must bring this to a close. The memory of Marsha, her positive attitude, her love of life and living each day to its fullest, her smile and strength are with me now. Whenever I find myself in the throes of a pity-party, I will evoke her spirit.

Thought For The Day

Our souls are hungry for meaning, for the sense that we have figured out how to live so that our lives matter, so that the world   will be at least a little bit different for our having passed through it… What frustrates us and robs us of joy is this absence of meaning… Does our being alive matter?

Harold S. Kushner

CHAPTER 41

DAY T+100

As hard as it is to believe, today I am 100 days out of transplant. Sometimes it feels a lifetime ago that Dr. Castro was hanging that bag of 'marinara' sauce from my IV pole. And at other times it seems like just yesterday. So vivid and emotional the memory.

Today is momentous in so many ways. I am out of the high risk period, though I must still take many precautions. I am feeling good other than the fatigue which sets in and forces me into long naps or early bedtimes. I have started working out, have been playing golf, riding my bike and walking two miles a day. Dr. Perales' raised eyebrows were the harbingers of what he was about to say. "And you wonder why you're tired. Your body is healing. You must take it slowly." Easy for him to say. His activity wasn't restricted for over a month. It is hard to sit still when I am feeling well. I was forced to sit still for too long.

Other milestones this past week include going out for a celebratory lunch at a local outdoor establishment for my first foray into restaurant eating. I still get strange looks when I tell the wait staff the restrictions they must follow when preparing my meal and serving it to me. But when I tell them that if they cannot accommodate me, I will have to eat elsewhere, they neither want to lose a customer nor can they afford a lawsuit of monstrous proportions.

I used shampoo for the first time the other day. My hair is starting to come back. I now have a goatee so that my baldness looks more like a true fashion statement than a chemo casualty. The hair on top of my head is just long enough for me to grab a hold of by pinching two fingernails together. I did take out my hairbrush from its resting place and looked in the mirror as I held it up to my head. Then I laughed at the absurdity of the image.

Walking Kristen down the aisle in July was the first goal I set for myself when I went in to the hospital. "Get through this successfully, Jim, and you will be able to go to her wedding," I thought. Today, I go shopping for the outfit I am to wear on her wedding day. And that is monumental. Today I also get to hear Sophia being adjudicated for her NYSSMA solo on the quarter bass, an instrument she started playing just 6 months ago and is already doing a level two solo. I have missed so many of these things in her life but no more. Her wedding date is now a long range goal of mine.

On Tuesday, Dr. Perales called with the results of last week's PET and CT scans. Hearing his voice is always a bit unnerving. Will he have good news or bad? I tried to focus on his words rather than the pounding in my chest. "Complete Remission". I made him repeat it to insure I had heard him correctly. Complete Remission. I had heard the words 'clear' and remission before, but never Complete Remission in the same breath. "Aaaaahhhhh!" echoed through the subsequent conversations with family and friends. But no greater "Aaaaahhhhh" was heard than from Nancy, who has shared this battle with me from mid-December 2006. And for her, it was a well-deserved "Aaaahhhhh".

Next week's bone marrow aspiration will tell whether my immune system is doing its job and given me a second shot at life. This will enable me to experience many more milestones and a lot more "Aaaahhhs"!

Thought For The Day

It's when ordinary people rise above the expectations and seize the opportunity that milestones truly are reached.

Mike Huckabee

Chapter 42

Day T+120

Today I am exactly four months out of transplant. February seems a lifetime ago and indeed it was. At times it has sped by and at others, dragged its ugly feet behind an IV pole decked with tubes and plastic bags of poison. But yesterday, at my bi-weekly appointment with Dr. Perales, whatever the last 4 months (in actuality, the last two and a half years) held for me, was well-worth enduring. I am now 100% the donor's bone marrow and her DNA as well. This means the graft took and I should not be susceptible to GVH disease and will no longer need IGIV infusions. The aspiration showed no cancer in my bone marrow. Meds have been reduced and I will be hitting from the forward tees from now on.

It becomes harder and harder to return to Sloan very two weeks. I see people suffering, stricken by this disease. I see people who are where I was over four months ago and I wonder if they really know what is in store for them. I sure didn't and it wasn't for lack of asking questions. It is a reminder and somewhat frightening to think back on.

Updates on the accidental family

Lisa is back in New Jersey, continuing her treatment there. She had to take a leave of absence from work as the side effects of the chemo and radiation incapacitate her significantly. She spent her 40th birthday alone and sick. Recently she returned to Hope Lodge to visit the people who care about her most and they report she is feeling and looking better. She calls often, but we have been playing phone tag a lot lately.

Stu, fresh off his interview with NBC which did a week-long series on "Facing Cancer", is still battling an infection for which he has been in and out of the hospital. Until that is cleared up, the surgery to remove his spleen which has swelled to seven times its size will have to be postponed.

Lew and Laurie find themselves back at Hope Lodge, merely three weeks after returning home with high hopes. Lew's counts have plummeted and the markers for Epstein-Barr virus are elevated. This setback has been devastating emotionally and physically for both.

Lee and Terry were released from 'bondage' a week ago and they are thriving. Lee was also interviewed by NBC but, alas, his mention of me somehow ended up on the cutting room floor. Since our appointments often coincide, we see each other more frequently than I do the others. Yesterday I had the good fortune to spend and hour or so catching up with them before he was called in. They have their sights set on Florida next winter season. Their place in Ft. Meyers is within an hour of my home in Sarasota and we plan to meet up after he has his long awaited hip replacement which started this all.

One final note for today. Four months ago I said to Dr. Perales, "Let me live long enough to walk my daughter down the aisle in July". For making that come true, I am eternally grateful to him and the transplant team at Sloan. These are milestones no parent should miss.

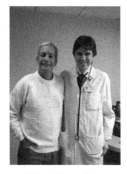 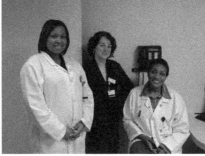 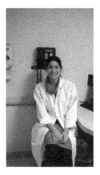

Dr. Perales and me   **Mary and Cecile with transplant nurses**

Thought For The Day

Our limitations and success will be based, most often
on our own expectations for ourselves. What the mind
dwells on, the body reacts to.

Denis Waitley

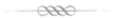

CHAPTER 43

DAY T+129

Today is my 63rd birthday. I greet the day with a mixture of emotions. Two and a half years ago when I was diagnosed in December of 2006, I was not sure if I would make it to my 61st birthday, let alone my 63rd. Today, I find myself looking forward to my 65th and 70th and beyond.

I never know what to say to people who ask what my status is. Do I say, "I have cancer"? Or do I say, "I had cancer"? My friend Susan, a cancer survivor herself, says, "I had cancer. I was treated for cancer. I am now cancer free." That has a nice ring to it. And while not a hollow ring, it does smack of a wee bit of arrogance. I guess arrogance is part of maintaining that strength needed to face this head on. But it is frightening in a way to let those words tumble out my mouth. What if it is not really true? It almost sounds like a smack down challenge to the disease. One I choose not to lose. What if I relapse though? Been there, done that three times already. Will I have jinxed myself? I certainly hope not and I certainly cannot afford to think that way.

A year ago today I spent my birthday alone a hospital room at Sloan puking my guts out from the side effects of the radiation I was receiving daily. It was terrifying and lonely. It showed me that no matter how much friends and family said they care and give their support, the bottom line is that we are really alone in all of this. When the lights go out at night and we lay in bed whether with someone or not, we are alone with our thoughts and our fears and our disease. One on one. It and me.

And it can be overwhelming.

During that hospital stay, my roommate, Tom Sawyer, of whom I have written previously, comes to mind today. He taught me so much about dignity, pride, self-esteem and survival. Thoughts of Tom make this less overwhelming. Unfortunately, I do not know what became of Tom, but my memory of him continues to serve as a constant reminder of who and what I want to be, today and forever.

Today I salute my fellow warriors. We are humbled by each other's setbacks but we rejoice and find strength in each other's victories.

Thought For The Day

Courage, it would seem, is nothing less than the power
to overcome danger, misfortune, fear, injustice, while
continuing to affirm inwardly that life with all its
sorrows is good; that everything is meaningful even if
in a sense beyond our understanding; and that there is
always tomorrow.

Dorothy Thomson

CHAPTER 44

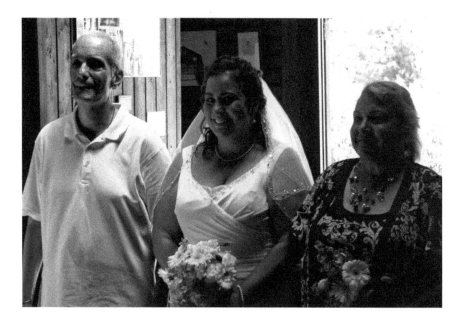

Today, I walked my daughter down the aisle. It was a very emotional moment as any father can attest. However, at the risk of sounding egotistical and self-important, this was more than just a special moment for her. I had been there before with Kristen's first marriage and my daughter Jamie's wedding and each was incredibly memorable. But today is different. When I first found out of their plans to marry, my concern was that I might not be able to participate in the joys of the day as I had a long hospital stay ahead of me and a battle with cancer I did not know I would survive. Not being able to walk Kristen down the aisle would have broken my heart, let alone my spirit if it did not take my life. I believe it was this that made me fight harder to be here today. It gave me purpose, a gift that all cancer patients need.

There must be a God in the heavens above. We get daily affirmations and even non-believers must admit that there is a higher power somewhere out there, regardless of how you envision him or her. It had rained throughout the months of May and June. Kristen had meticulously and with great attention to detail, planned a beach wedding. All was under her control. All, that is, except the weather. As the day drew close all eyes and ears were on the weather forecast. At first long range, then 10 day, then 5 day. Still there was no guarantee, even if Lee Goldberg or Al Roker said it would be nice day on July 6th. We all have made our smart aleck remarks about many a weatherman's ability to do his/her job.

But faith is another thing altogether and Doppler 4000 be damned. Today was the most perfect day for an outdoor wedding — sunny, warm, gentle breezes, glass-like water conditions and low humidity for those who have hair cares. I remember those days.

The bride and her attendants were whisked away via private sailboat across the Great South Bay to the wedding destination — a small chapel on Davis Park on the Fire Island National Seashore. The groom, his attendants and the rest of the wedding guests were ferried and the day began smoothly.

From the moment I took my place next to Kristen and her mother, I fought to suppress the great upheaval of emotion. Through somewhat clenched teeth, my daughter strained the words, "Don't you start crying!" I fought to obey her wishes then took hold of her arm. She said, "I'm all right, Dad. I'm pretty steady." Little did she know that I was taking her arm to steady myself not her. And so we, the three of us, made the walk to the waiting groom.

And they were married and it was good.

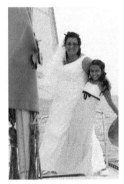
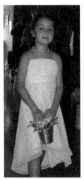
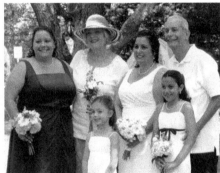

Kristen and   **Mykayla**   **Jamie, Nancy Mykayla Kristen,**
Sophia   **Sophia and Dad**

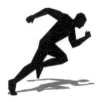

Thought For The Day

At times our own light goes out and is rekindled by
a spark from another person. Each of us has cause to
think with deep gratitude of those who have lighted the
flame within us.

Albert Schweitzer

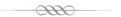

CHAPTER 45

DAYS T+142 AND T+143

What follows is what we cancer patients who have gone through treatment and emerged victorious, in "complete remission", fear the most. It is a constant worry. "Ooh I have a hang nail. Maybe it's finger cancer". Not to make light of this but these are the bizarre places our minds go to. At times we are able to put them on the back burner and get on with our lives, functioning normally. And then at others, it comes roaring back into our consciousness often unexpectedly, echoing, reverberating, screaming.

The following are transcripts of emails sent yesterday and today between Lew and me. He is one day behind me in transplant time so we are in a sense "cell mates" and I have a strong connection to him because of our coincidental timetables:

(note: I do not use capitals in emails)

hey lew,
got an email from laurie yesterday and she said that you were going to be up at sloan today for an unscheduled visit. i hope everything is all right. when you can, let me know how you're doing. sorry to hear that you had to make this unscheduled trip. the wedding was beautiful. i am so thankful on so many levels.

Jim,

We are so happy that the wedding went so well. We did go to Sloan today. A blood smear earlier this week indicated blast cells. Sloan confirmed today that the leukemia is back and I will likely have to go through induction chemo and another transplant all starting very soon. Will get more details tomorrow. Needless to say, we are very upset.

I'll let you know as we know more. Lew

lew,

when i got home last night i read your email and could not find the words to express how i felt and so i could not, did not write back. this morning i woke up and am still at a loss for what to say. i am very upset for you. i cannot imagine what you and laurie must be going through right now. i don't know how i would handle it. just know that my prayers are with you both. i hope that you can get through this next battle without the scars of the first and it will be successful. nancy is likewise devastated by this and she sends her love and prayers as well. please keep us updated when you can.

jim

Jim,

thank you so much for your thoughts and prayers. I am having a tough time today, waiting to get direction from Sloan. I should hear later today. I'll let you know

Lew

And so it goes. Lew's words echoed and reverberated all night and all through the day. I know. I don't have the same cancer. I know. I don't have the same doctor. I know. My body reacts differently than anybody's else's body. But I am cancer patient. I have been treated just as Lew has. I have been told I am in complete remission as I suspect Lew was. And I was told that I am 100% my donor's DNA, bone marrow and blood type. I am sure Lew was on or close to those numbers or his doctor would never have let him go home to Maryland. Is this all the medical profession can give us — false hope? Is it a reminder that nothing is definite?

Lew will be re-admitted to Sloan this coming Tuesday. Then the pre-testing will begin, another port will be put in and chemo administered to get him back into remission. Then he will either get a full transplant or what they call a boost or T cell infusion. Mercifully, Lew's bother was the original donor and another does not have to be found. The doctors are confident that because he did so well the first time he should tolerate this equally as well. In Laurie's words, "It is so weird to hear that when it felt so difficult to us."

And the words continue to echo and reverberate.. First time, second time …. how many more times. One could make a case that having been through all this before, it should be easier the second time, knowing what to expect. "You handled it so well the first time". Ironic, no?

Echoes.

Flashbacks to the events of the last six months. A friend of mine calls me the 'poster boy for stem cell transplants' and while I'm flattered by the title the thought of being hooked up to 10, 11, 12 bags of fluid, getting chemo, enduring the side effects of GVHD, being awakened at 4 AM to have vitals taken, and being kept isolation for four or more weeks makes me want to relinquish my crown in favor of never having to experience any of this again.

Reverberations.

And yet what is the alternative. The return of the cancer is only part of the battle, deciding what to do next is another whole ballgame.

Screams.

The trials continue for Lew and Laurie . The latest from her is that he is struggling with this. He is "depressed sad and teary" — her words. I can only imagine. He does not feel well and the pain the in his back, which he has never had before, is from the return of the leukemia. During the summer of 2007 in relapse mode, I experienced excruciating back pain. I had to be taken to the hospital where they damn near-on killed me with pain killers which shut down my respiratory system and my ability to swallow. No one told me it might be a return of the lymphoma. I understand, in some measure, what Lew is experiencing.

The brain is an amazing organ. It works in such, ok it's a cliche, mysterious ways. Mine is particularly bizarre. It forges links between things that most people would never connect. It is skilled at avoiding pain and trying to make itself laugh at the ironies of life. At times like this when I find it difficult to cope with what is happening around me, my brain somehow magnetizes the absurdities in the universe and attracts them into my conscious world.

On July 8th an article about a man in New Jersey who drowned in a vat of melted chocolate appeared on the Internet. The following is a reproduction of that article:

Man Falls Into a Vat of Chocolate, Dies.

Camden, N.J. (July 8) Authorities say a man died after falling into a vat of melted chocolate in a New Jersey processing plant. The Camden County prosecutor's office identified the victim as 29 year old Vincent Smith II of Camden. He was a temporary worker at Cocoa Services Inc. plant.

The accident happened Wednesday morning as Smith was loading chocolate into a vat where it is melted and mixed before being shipped elsewhere to be made into candy."

When I read this article, I started to laugh, not unlike the Mary Tyler Moore episode of "Chuckles the Clown" in which Chuckles dressed as a peanut meets his untimely death at the hands or rather the feet of a rogue elephant during a parade. Everyone, Murray, Ted, Lou, Sue Ann could not control their laughter at Chuckle's unexpected and absurd demise. Mary chastised them all for their insensitivity. But at the services for Chuckles, it is she who loses control and cannot stop herself from laughing while the others become serious and introspective. The point of the episode obviously was that our laughter anesthetizes pain and loss. It stops us from hurting even if only momentarily. And so it was with me when I read the article about the tragic death of Vincent Smith. I laughed thinking only of the lyrics of an old Smothers Brothers song, which had been hidden in the dark recesses of my mind, cobwebbed over, just waiting for the right moment to be dusted off and called upon.

The lyrics of which follow:

Tom (singing): I fell into a vat of chocolate. I fell into a vat of chocolate.
Dick (singing): What'd you do when you fell in the chocolate?
Both: La dee doo dum la dee doo dum day.

Tom (singing): I yelled fire when I fell into the chocolate.

Dick (annoyed, singing): Why'd you yell fire when you fell into the chocolate?

Tom: I yelled fire cause no one would help me if I yelled chocolate.

Laughter is the universal language transcending all barriers. It's known to be an instinctual survival tool, which reduces interpersonal stress, even more than an intellectual response to a joke. Alison Stormwolf says, "Laughter is essential to our overall well-being. It strengthens the immune system, releases the 'feel good' endorphins and shows on our faces eventually making us so much more beautiful and approachable. Those who try to rid their faces of laughter lines do themselves a great disservice"

And so I laughed at the irony that if the man who really had fallen into the vat of chocolate had only yelled "fire" he would not have perished.

And I laughed again, if only to shield myself against the hurt.

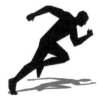

Thought For The Day

Laughter and tears are both responses to frustration and exhaustion.. I myself prefer to laugh since there is less cleaning up to do afterward.

Kurt Vonnegut

CHAPTER 46

Today I am four days shy of being a half year out of transplant. Frequently, the time has gone quickly but in re-reading some of these journal entries, it seems eons ago that this process began. Yesterday I had my scheduled sixth month CT scan. I am sure that no matter how many days or years past transplant I get, that week preceding a scan of any type, will produce the same feeling. I awoke this morning and realized that waiting for the phone to ring with the results would be useless and stressful, so I tried somewhat successfully to make the time fly by going to the chiropractor and running pedestrian errands. When I returned there were no messages. However, the phone did ring several times but for the most part the calls were from family and friends wanting to hear the good news. I hurried them off the phone to keep the lines clear for Dr. Perales' call. Cancer patients who are waiting for results should have a hot line installed for that express purpose. I know there is call waiting, but I don't have it. I waited for what I thought was an appropriate amount of time for the call to come, before I took the proverbial bull by the horns and called for the results myself. Of course, them's that answer the phone in a physician's office are not qualified, or to be more exact, not permitted, to give results. Dr. Perales knows my anxiety levels rise while waiting for results and he called back almost immediately. Scans were clear and Dr. Perales was happy, but no more than I. I am now free of stress and anxiety until the next scan.

Unfortunately, this post is not without a downside. Lew's condition has worsened. The leukemia is still present in his spine and the chemo injections designed to combat it are not working as well as had been hoped. His fungal pneumonia has taken a turn for the worse and he cannot walk or even pivot on his feet He is sleeping a lot and this is not good. According to Laurie, Lew has chosen to take control of the only thing he can control now and that is who visits him. He has not allowed even his parents who have come up from Florida to come into his room. To Lew, this does not portend good things. He is accepting nothing less than success. He has, however, signed a DNR authorization. Laurie is caught between Lew's wishes, those of his parents and her own. In her words, "Sometimes I can't even breathe, my heart is broken and I am angry at everything imaginable."

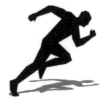

Thought For The Day

⎯⎯⎯⎯◊◊◊⎯⎯⎯⎯

Miracles are not contrary to nature, but are only
contrary to what we know about nature.

St. Augustine

EPILOGUE

DAY T+180 BUT RIGHT NOW, THAT NO LONGER MATTERS

I am writing this to honor my friend, Lew Zagar, who lost his battle with leukemia tonight at 7:20 PM. I cannot begin to describe the sense of loss and emptiness his passing leaves. I received an email from Laurie this morning which said the doctors felt that anyone wanting to visit should do so today. I knew I could not live at peace had I not gone to see him at the hospital. Today, I met Lew's parents, his brother and sister, Linda, and I saw Laurie.

How does one maintain hope when all that you are told speaks to the contrary. Yet none of these people had given up hope. And Lew kept fighting the insurmountable odds facing him. I am grateful that I was allowed to go into his room and speak with him directly. Although I had to wear a mask, gloves and gown for my own protection as well as Lew's, it was good to stand close to his bedside. His morphine induced haze broke for a few minutes and he opened his eyes, recognized me and smiled. He even managed to thank me for visiting. I held his hand for a moment and then quietly left the room, fighting the swell of emotions surging inside me, as he gently slipped back to sleep. His family sat vigil outside the room. Their faces and the touch of Lew's hand linger.

There are no words of comfort to speak at time such as this. Everything seems patently insignificant. I will continue to honor Lew's memory by my actions and by striving to live my life to its fullest, never taking for granted even one minute or one person in it.

I know that at Hope Lodge, Lew, Lee and I were the Three Musketeers of the 12th floor kitchen. We engaged in verbal swordplay to amuse ourselves, to fight off our fears and to talk of things other than cancer. Our verbal parrying and thrusting fostered our healing. We were all in the same boat, three men, who under other circumstances, might never have become friends. But we had a bond that drew us together to share information, insights and funny stories. We were able to defend ourselves both individually and as a band of brothers against the emotional and physical forces that sought to destroy us. We kept each other grounded. Lew, whose rapier like wit, like a paper cut that you don't realize happened until you see the thin red line of blood, took great joy in and got much mileage out of my female DNA status. I can still see his bright blue eyes and the sly, subtle upturn of his lips, knowing he had drawn first blood with a Zagar Zinger.

Tonight my sadness is for the loss of a family member and the grief of his parents, Laurie, his daughter and family.

Lew may you be at peace, out of pain and free from care. Look down on all of us kindly and keep Laurie under the umbrella of your love.

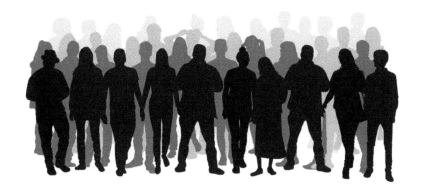

Thought For The Day

———◌∞◌———

There are a million, and none suffice.

Afterword

Writing this book has been liberating. It has taken 15 years to come to grips with this and process it all. I spent so much time thinking of how this disease would affect others and tried to protect them, that taking care of myself became secondary.

In his book <u>Illusions</u>, Richard Bach writes:

> There is
> no such thing as a problem
> without a gift for you
> in its hands.
> You seek problems
> because you need
> their gifts.

I did not seek out cancer. Trust me on this one. But it found me. And in its wake left me with several gifts. Yes, gifts. Those words have been met with strange looks from friends and family. The problems cancer challenged me with held a multitude of awakenings. I learned how to prioritize things in my life and to prioritize myself which, in essence, was my way of healing. It made me leave behind all the baggage I had been carrying for so many years which had made me weary without my even being aware how weary. It has made me accept YOLO as a mantra — You Only Live Once — because I know and appreciate the transitory nature of life and fully enjoy what I have, and not what I have lost. And there have been losses. But those losses have made me a kinder person because of the kindness shown to me by friends and family and yes, even strangers.

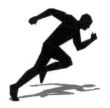

Thought For The Day

You can't wait until life isn't hard anymore
before you decide to be happy.

Jane Marczewski
Nightbirde

Along with Lew's passing, it must be noted that Terry, Lee's wife, was diagnosed with lung cancer which metastasized to her brain. Terry lost her battle in July a year and a half ago. Her loss is as tragic to me as Lew's passing. Ironic, that caretaker and patient switched roles. Terry who was Lee's caretaker became the patient, and Lee her caretaker. I do not know how Lee has summoned the courage and the strength to go through this and emerge even stronger. I spoke with him recently and he is surviving. Better than surviving — thriving. We plan to meet this spring. This is for you, Lee.

Grief

I had my own notion of grief
I thought it was a sad time
That followed the death of someone you love
And you had to push through it
To get to the other side.
But I'm learning there is no other side.
There is no pushing through.
But rather,
There is absorption.
Adjustment.
Acceptance.
And grief is not something that you complete.
But rather you endure.
Grief is not a task to finish.
And move on.
But an element of yourself —
An alteration of your being.
A new way of seeing,
A new definition of self.

On another noted entirely February 17 of this year, 2022 marks my 13th re-birthday. It is worthy of celebration. But today I celebrate my dear friend, Tom, and his wife Barbara, who never forget my "birthday". He makes a special point every year to celebrate this day with me. They take me to lunch, often accompanied by our friends Ray and Sue and Bob and Lenore. They make me feel visible with their remembrance.

Couple these two wonderful friends with my cousin, Bobbie, who without fail has sent me a birthday card every February for 13 years.

I am most fortunate to be remembered after so much time has passed. Some of us, along with all our experiences are not remembered now that we are "healthy". It is so meaningful to me to be remembered, to be recognized for what I have endured.

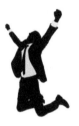

Resources

American Cancer Society
    1-800-227-2345
    http://www.cancer.org/docroot/home/index.asp

Memorial Sloan-Kettering
    1275 York Ave
    NYC, NY 10065
    212-639-2000 1-646-888-4740
    http://mskcc.org. mskcc/html/19409 Post Treatment Center

Hope Lodge There are many throughout the country
    132 W. 32nd St
    NYC, NY 10001
    1-800-227-2345

Leukemia Lymphoma Society
    1-800-482-TEAM
    1-800-955-4572

National Institute of Health (NIH)
    9000 Rockville Pike
    Bethesda, MD 20892
    301-496-4000

Cancer Resource Services (insurance coverage)
    ℅ OptimumHealth Care Solutions
    PO Box 30758
    Salt Lake City, UT 84130

Moffitt Cancer Center
    12902 USF Magnolia Drive
    Tampa, FL 336127
    1-813-745-4673

National Cancer Institute
    http://www.cancer.gov/
    1-800-4-CANCER

National Coalition for Cancer Survivorship
    http//www. canceradvocacy.org/
    1-877-CCS.YES

Livestrong
    www.livestrong.org
    1-866-235-7205

CancerCare
    http://www.cancercare.org/
    1-800-813-HOPE

Blog
    caringbridge.org

CPSIA information can be obtained
at www.ICGtesting.com
Printed in the USA
LVHW070044270822
726990LV00007B/312